CULTIVATING WELLNESS IN BLACK NEIGHBORHOODS

Rashni Stanford and Mel Brown

CULTIVATING WELLNESS IN BLACK NEIGHBORHOODS

Establishing Philadelphia's Deep Space Mind 215 Cooperative

Disability Studies

Collection Editor

Damian Mellifont

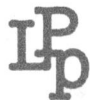

LᴘP

First published in 2025 by Lived Places Publishing

The authors and editor have made every effort to ensure the accuracy of the information contained in this publication, but assume no responsibility for any errors, inaccuracies, inconsistencies, or omissions. Likewise, every effort has been made to contact copyright holders. If any copyright material has been reproduced unwittingly and without permission, the publisher will gladly receive information enabling them to rectify any error or omission in subsequent editions.

British Library Cataloguing in Publication Data
A CIP record for this book is available from the British Library.

ISBN: 9781916704886 (pbk)
ISBN: 9781916704909 (ePDF)
ISBN: 9781916704893 (ePUB)

The right of Rashni Stanford and Mel Brown to be identified as the Authors of this work has been asserted by them in accordance with the Copyright, Design and Patents Act 1988.

Cover design by Fiachra McCarthy
Book design by Rachel Trolove of Twin Trail Design
Typeset by Newgen Publishing, UK

Lived Places Publishing
P.O. Box 1845
47 Echo Avenue
Miller Place, NY 11764

www.livedplacespublishing.com

Abstract

Cultivating Wellness In Black Neighborhoods: Establishing Philadelphia's Deep Space Mind 215 Cooperative is a collection of experiences and emerging practices and frameworks in neighborhood mental health and Black care work as developed by members of Deep Space Mind 215 Co-operative, alongside neighbors who work in partnership with DSM215 in the city of Philadelphia. Deep Space Mind 215 was formed in the midst of the global COVID-19 pandemic, during the political unrest following the wake of racialized, ableist police violence both locally and nationally, when many fissures, hypocrisies, and meltdowns in all sectors of the care, social service, and healthcare industries were laid bare. It is against this backdrop that *Cultivating Wellness in Black Neighborhoods* documents and contextualizes the collective's work. This book collects personal accounts of mental health recovery journeys, institutionalization, and survivorship; emerging grassroots practice and praxis development informed by DSM215's first community projects, afrofuturism, and disability justice; archival material from local partnerships; and interviews with neighbors who have collaborated with DSM215 to build collaborative spaces for wellness, community care, and self-determination. The collection reminds readers, students, care workers and mental health professionals, and survivors of institutional systems that those living with mental health challenges have the capacity to bring humanizing care to local neighborhoods, and that local wisdom in the form of peership, survivorship, and Black and Indigenous ancestral traditions are indispensable assets in the work to increase wellness and joy in Black communities.

Keywords

Lived experience, invisible illness, community mental health, mental health harm reduction, misogynoir, complex trauma, state-sanctioned violence, mad afrofuturisms, Black healing experiences, ancestral healing, disability justice

Contents

Content warning

In this book, we discuss our lived experiences of navigating psychosis and the Western psychiatric industrial complex which includes the following difficult or triggering content dealing with themes of

- family violence, death;
- suicide, sucidality;
- personal accounts of self-harm, substance abuse, psychosis;
- ableism and white supremacy culture, misogynoir;
- psychiatric industrial complex, detainment, institutionalization;
- child sexual abuse, sexual violence;
- criminal and juvenile legal systems, detention, incarceration.

We made our best attempt to warn readers before subsequent chapters that address the aforementioned themes. Please do what is necessary to have emotional safety and care while continuing. If you or anyone you know is struggling with suicidality, please call 988, or for more resources, specifically LGBTQIA+, visit https://www.thetrevorproject.org/get-help/.

Learning objectives

1.   Defining key terms and integrating real-life accounts related to the Western medical industrial complex.

2.   Understanding the long-term effects of complex trauma in Black communities beyond the dichotomy of micro- versus macro- frameworks.

3.   Understanding the significant impact of community wellness as a means of mental health harm reduction.

4.   Understanding of real-life examples of community-led resilience and self-determination.

5.   Capacity to provide examples of how madness leads to new approaches and methodologies for community healing.

Foreword

Rasheedah Philips

We all have that one secret we haven't told our parents—the one thing that, if they knew, would shatter their world. Maybe they've discovered it and chosen to ignore it, or perhaps they've been waiting for you to reveal it. It's also possible that they remain blissfully unaware, forever innocent. But is your secret a black hole or a white hole? Is it a simple yes, no, or maybe? Is it like the shake of a magic 8-ball or the shuffle of a fortune teller's deck, revealing glimpses of fate as a game of chance?

Fate, it seems, is always just beyond our grasp. It is like a hand drawing itself, an eye that cannot see itself unless it looks in the mirror—and even then, it's not a true reflection but a reversal, an inside-out view of the self along the z-axis. This disorienting perspective allows us to get lost or even switch selves with another world. Perhaps this is how I ended up here—maybe I tumbled out of a mirror, as I had always stared into the second-floor bathroom mirror as a child. The small, silver-framed mirror would captivate me for minutes on end until I no longer recognized myself, until I stood on the brink of sanity, feeling almost, almost gone. But did I truly go somewhere? Maybe. I felt strange all the time, but when did that strangeness begin? I recall feeling relatively normal until I was around six when I was first touched by someone I knew. We were watching TV after my Grandmom and his dad had fallen asleep. He was a few years older than me, and the

TV was just gray squiggly lines on Channel 7 until, at around 2 a.m., the commercials for 900 hotlines began.

From a young age, I struggled with depression, long before I had the language for it or understood that I had been a victim of sexual violence. My first "real" suicide attempt occurred nearly a decade later. My boyfriend at the time, who was with me when I locked myself in the bathroom and took a handful of pills, took care of the baby and called the ambulance, and I ended up in a hospital bed, drinking a cup full of charcoal. That day opened several paths for me, like the mirror world I had stumbled into a decade earlier. There were worlds and possibilities beyond the immediate reality of my existence, and I made the choice to get better, to live, to follow the unexpected path.

Part of the reason why cycles of poverty and trauma perpetuate and repeat is because the stories behind the statistics are rendered invisible, go unacknowledged, or are manipulated to suit particular agendas. When our stories and our truths go untold and unshared, the cycles of trauma are bound to repeat, with no space or time given to evaluate one's journey and shift course. Understanding how trauma and post-traumatic stress can connect or disconnect us from our pasts, and the ways in which human behavior, in the aggregate, can influence an entire community or city, or how historical events, such as slavery or war, transform our communities in such a way that it displaces us completely from those events and their sources. We not only see ourselves reflected in these stories; we see our mothers and our fathers, our sisters and our brothers, our neighbors and our friends. That means that the work of healing extends beyond the individual to begin to reverse the vicious and destructive cycles that our communities have fallen into due to institutions which systematically deny the right to life, liberty, justice, shelter, service, and good health.

Black madness, and the accompanying states of Black mental wholeness and expression, are essential to both Afrofuturism and the broader project of Black survival. Afrofuturism harnesses the radical imagination to envision futures where Black people are liberated from systemic oppression. Black madness, as a response to and product of these systemic pressures, acts as a catalyst for creative expression and innovation, pushing us to reimagine reality and explore possibilities that extend beyond the limitations of the present. Scholars like Therí A. Pickens have examined how Black neurodiversities challenge conventional temporal frameworks, offering a perspective that disrupts linear time and opens up spaces for radical hope and the wild imagination of new realities (Pickens, 2019). This is not merely a theoretical exercise but a lived experience that transforms how we understand and engage with time.

In my personal journey, depression and anxiety have often manifested as a dread of the linear future—a fear that events would unfold in their worst possible form. This fear stems from a traditional view of time as a straightforward progression from cause to effect, where the future is a mere extension of the present. Yet, as I delved into time, community, and quantum physics over the years, I came to recognize the limitations of this linear perspective. Black madness, with its unique temporalities and spatialities, offers an alternative. It disrupts the linear flow of time and transforms predetermined outcomes into a realm of potential possibilities.

This transformative potential aligns with Black Quantum Futurism, a theory and practice that envisions time not as a rigid continuum but as a dynamic, fluid entity shaped by the interconnectedness of past, present, and future. In the spirit of quantum mechanics, where particles exist in multiple states and outcomes are probabilistic rather than deterministic, Black madness offers a quantum-like understanding of time. It reveals that the future is not a predetermined path but a landscape of infinite possibilities, shaped by our collective imagination and radical hope.

The insights of Black madness scholars such as Sami Schalk further illuminate this perspective. Schalk explores how Black neurodiversities and disability provide a lens to see beyond the constraints of linear time, creating spaces for new, liberating temporal experiences (Schalk, 2018). These experiences are not confined by the oppressive structures that seek to limit Black existence but offer a vision for transformative change.

Embracing Black madness allows us to tap into a deep well of radical hope and imagination, enabling us to envision and strive for new realities that transcend the limitations of the present while embracing a vision of the future that is expansive and inclusive of diverse Black experiences. Black madness, therefore, is not merely a condition to be managed but a source of profound temporal agency and creative potential. This perspective not only challenges the status quo but also offers a visionary framework for creating just and equitable realities for Black communities.

#

The extreme fringes of life, characterized by instability and the fragility of sanity, serve as spaces of not only immense pressure but also incredible innovation. Historically, Black people have had to innovate to survive, creating new cultural, social, and technological practices in response to systemic oppression. These innovations often arise from the necessity of navigating and resisting these oppressive structures. The experiences of Black madness act as a bridge to other realities, offering insights and knowledge that enhance and transform our current reality. The concept of moving between different states of being and knowing resonates with Afrofuturist modes of time travel, alternate dimensions, and speculative futures.

The survival of Black communities hinges on resilience and adaptability. Exploring Black madness and mental wholeness reveals how Black people have resisted and adapted to oppressive systems, creating resilient communities that endure and evolve. Understanding Black madness as a form of temporal and creative agency allows us to challenge the pathologization of Black experiences and reframe them as sources of power and innovation. This shift empowers us to define our own narratives and envision new futures.

Being on the extreme fringes of life positions Black people at the edge of space and time, where conventional boundaries blur and new possibilities emerge. This liminal space is fertile ground for Black creative and futurist thought, which seeks to transcend current limitations and imagine collective futures where Black people are thriving. Within these fringes, innovation occurs, breaking through to other realities and bringing back transformative ways of being, existing, and knowing. Within these fringes, we are affirmed that Black madness is not an aberration but a profound expression of resistance and resilience. It embodies the capacity to imagine and create new worlds, where Black people are free from systemic oppression haunting our futures and able to thrive in our full humanity. Embracing Black madness as a source of temporal and creative power is essential for envisioning and building these new futures.

The path to change and healing is not an easy one, for it requires collaboration and a dismantling of deep-rooted cycles of trauma. It is a journey that encompasses all levels of existence—from the particle level to the whole self to the communal to the global to the universal. We cannot make this journey alone. Telling our stories and speaking our truths allow us to practically explore the ways in which our collective and personal pasts continue to affect us and share sustainable solutions to breaking cycles of trauma. This book contains the truth, words, hopes, dreams, lessons, experiences, wisdom, and stories of those who are best positioned to speak on it and identify the solutions.

Introduction

This book outlines the early years of Deep Space Mind 215 Co-operative and its projects in the city of Philadelphia concerning the humanization and inclusion of those with lived experience of mental health challenges, neurodiversities, and confinement in institutions in local leadership around community care and health innovation. DSM215 has utilized a variety of community interventions to connect with and continue ongoing dialogue and shared action with neighbors, including afrofuturism, art-based interventions, restorative circle practice, psychoeducation, and peer support.

We will lead you through our lived experiences as long-time mental health and social service workers, community organizers, and survivors of institutionalization and psychiatric experiences. This will serve as the foundation from which DSM215 co-founders Rashni Stanford and Mel Brown bring you our frame-works toward Black disability justice, Mad pride, and centering peership and lived experience while building care alternatives to carceral systems in Black communities.

Next, we will discuss DSM215's recent historical context and emerging frameworks and solutions around Black mental health, community care, and a radical reimagining of what community mental health looks like for those who have seen how institutional systems tear Black communities apart, rather than restore safety and humanity.

Then we will hear from our neighbor's voices and the experiences that have colored our collaborative work, as well as how DSM215's way of working has begun impacting our local network.

Lastly, we share with you our Syllabus and Archive, including exercises from our workshops, archival materials from our partnerships, and resources for collective care.

We have included discussion questions with each chapter, meant to challenge the reader to look for ways to apply tenets of centering lived experience, local history, and destigmatizing madness and radical imagination in service of real life, effective and humanizing care for those suffering from mental health challenges.

#

Thank you to our community: DSM215 Autumn 2024

#

We at DSM215 acknowledge and recognize all of the Philadelphians, all the young people, elders, children, all of the animals, spirits, and ancestors—all the madness, creativity, and imagination. Thank you for the struggle, the mess, and the not-so-salient successes. And thank you for the belly laughs, shared joy, and shared grief.

We are grateful for the young people at YASP who shared their sorrow with us on the morning of a fallen comrade's funeral. And those who celebrated birthdays and low days at our workshops and training. We are grateful for the jams, jellies, and tinctures our neighbors made and shared with us, and for the kindness and warmth bestowed upon us by our elders at Pentridge Children's Garden. We thank the groundhogs, cats, hummingbirds, catbirds, and cardinals. We thank the porgy of the Delaware Bay and the jellyfish of the Chesapeake. We thank the black squirrels of Detroit that dart around Mama Myrtle's mushrooms at Freedom Freedom Farm. We thank French for growing with us.

> *Thank you to the space for radical imagination provided by comrades at Black Quantum Futurist Collective, Community Futures Lab, Black Womxn's Time Camp, and Metropolarity. For Joshua Glenn of Youth Art & Self Empowerment project, Sul'Yah Williams, Jimmy Mao, Chynna Rogers, Dominique "Rem'mie" Fells, and the beloved gardeners of Pentridge Children's Garden.*

Neighborhood partners:
- Creative Resilience Youth [CRY]
- Young Artist Program [YAP]
- Youth Art and Self-Empowerment Project [YASP]
- Philly Homes 4 Youth Coalition
- UrbEd
- PhillyCam
- Eddie's House
- The Philadelphia Rent Control Coalition
- Hook and Loop
- Restorative Cities Initiative
- The Dynamic Justice Collective
- Metropolitan Christian Council of Philadelphia

- House of Umoja
- Neighbors/communities of people (e.g., consumers and workers within local systems, those with lived experience of foster care, homelessness, mental health, etc.)

Green Space Partners:

- Gente de Tierra Collective
- Join Heinz Wildlife Center
- Urban Creators
- One Art Community Center

Press Partners:

- Lived Places Publishing
- Resolve Philly
- The Appeal

National:

- National Council of Elders
- Feedom Freedom Farm Detroit
- PolicyLink
- Afrofuture Youth

Institutional supporters:

- Philadelphia Area Cooperative Alliance
- Villanova Legal Clinic

1
Experiences

In this chapter DSM215 co-founders present lived experience of mental health challenges, including but not limited to intergenerational struggle with suicidality, interpersonal struggle, the effects of racial capitalism, chronic subjugation of Black people's time and labor. CW: Suicidality, intergenerational trauma, sexual violence, institutional violence, C-PTSD

#

A personal account of suicidality and time subjugation - Mel Brown

This is dedicated to loved ones who've transitioned to another space-time on their own terms. I love and cherish all that you had to give, suffered through, in transition to the other side of "things." This chapter is hard for me to write but I'm gonna make my best attempt to explain the thresholds of my body, time, psychosis, and my flirtations with the great abyss that is death, which we all must face alone.

For those who stare into the sun

My mother was in marital bliss, which would take me and my youngest older brother from a western coastal shoreside of the

Bay Area to a vast landlocked place called Saint Louis, Missouri. I was in the third grade and joined my peers late in the year, and I remember being excited about snow. Later that year, there was a total lunar eclipse. As a class we covered the basics, the transition of the moon, made our pinhole eye glasses, but for whatever reason I chose to stare into the sun. After being told many tall tales of the hazards of doing so, I insisted on experiencing it for myself. I was curious about many things at a young age, with the understanding that there was more to things, often searching for elsewhere, another place, or maybe somewhere beyond the tears of my mother, and her mother, and her mother (fades out).

I am named after my grandmother, who I never met. Her name was Elizabeth. I learned more about her in depth when I was pregnant at 19 with my first child. Heavy with birth, I asked my mother, "what was she like?," and "why was I named after her?" Comforting my questioning mind, laying beside me, my mother recited all the ways she witnessed her mother's beauty, poise, and how I so much resemble her. Elizabeth died unexpectedly, which was always referred to but never explicitly explained; her death was a mystery to me and my siblings. Heartbrokenly my grandmother took her life. I pictured my mother with soft skin, holding my eldest brother to her breast, at her mother's funeral asking myself, "Was she relieved that she didn't have to care for her mother's grief any longer?" Wondering if my grandmother also stared into the abyss? Forever changed, misunderstood?

Having grown up in the church, my obsession with heaven and hell at an early age forced me to excel in memorizing my bible verses, holding on tight to the warnings of being a bad person wishing "if only I could be good." Thinking the only way to be good was through suffering like the character Job from the Old Testament because everyone who was righteous had a "cross" to bear, which was just a biblical way of saying that everyone had their own individualized suffering they had to do in this lifetime. This life was your own personal hell, and no, you can't skip ahead by your own hand or you go to eternal hell and that was forever. My mental health began to fail in a new way by the time I was in junior high. Overwhelmed and worried, when I should've been a carefree preteen, I remember the walls of my bedroom, the stiffness of my small body, being perceived as too much, with breasts that developed too fast. I wanted so badly to escape my body and the suicidal ideation came and never left.

I'm in college, organizing other women, protesting police violence in the Shaw neighborhood of Saint Louis in the early 2000s, fervently reading radical Black feminist prose when I reach Ntozake Shange's *For Colored Girls Who've Considered Suicide When the Rainbow Is Enuf*. I was comforted once again with words describing myself, but this time Ntozake. She comforted me, reminding me that this so-called reality, or place, was never meant to hold the first version of queer, described as other than, or Black femme (Shange, 1997).

Time subjugation madness

My pathology relieves me of a certain type of fixed time or the kind of time that muscle memory relies on for its retention. Monotonous time, like how long it takes for you to walk to school every morning, or get to the bus stop from your stoop, it's the kind of time that's the same every time. But for me, there's a faintness that's between here (real time) and some other time. I slip often between the two, where there's no distinction of beginning or end. My brain is busted, with no first memory, my memories forever to be in a flux that my body struggles to keep up with. In my time of being in that "other place," or institutionalized, the stillness of time is what I remember.

When memory is brittle and slippery, I sometimes go somewhere, or maybe in between, but we've heard that before. The periphery or the upside down, the sunken place. I am here but absent from now. The temporal space, somewhere in between, requires a stretching of place. How can I be here and there without overextending the limits of my body, or "spirit." We know that under systems of violent status quo, or white hegemony, being in two places at once is a disservice to productivity because those subjugated should remain tethered to (real-time) production.

I oscillate between time dysfunction and being time poor.

Poor people live in a linear dichotomy of time.

Poor people die slow deaths, waiting for the money to come, living check to check, living the repetitive 9 to 5 time.

Poor people die fast deaths when tricking time, insert lessons of quick money, and early deaths.

The only way out is through, in this case, a lie.

I've been making my best attempt to write this email for a few weeks. I understand why, I've come to the conclusion that when one's dreams are directly opposed to the reality of resources there's an undeniable stopgap. I ask myself often, how could I be so privileged to dream?

In my journal, I write,

....how could I imagine freedom while living in time captivity, of a geo-social-political landscape of terror?

Yet I am inspired to live and die with dignity, in these last days of late-stage capitalism. I recognize that this system ensures that I will die working, to live. When I think of radical time liberation, I think of the Igbo people in 1803 who marched into the sea chained together.... and how time stopped—on the shore of St. Simon's Island, they turned their backs to captivity, to a lifetime sentence of servitude[1].

I'm here, now, knowing our children will go to fight yet another war, just like our fathers, and their fathers. I am inconsolable, how could I hold tight to me what has never truly belonged to me? With no access to object permanence, or a future.

Furthermore, I write,

> No one is coming to save you. Not your father or brother, not the church man, or the earnest man, not the one who sings to you.

My interrogation of suicidality under generational ableist capitalism not only offers liberation in death but also serves as a warning for us to abolish the whelms of late-stage capitalism, while some of us are still "living."

#

Mad Black time cures for institutional trauma - Rashni Stanford

A Temporal Study of Institutional Trauma,

I remember the old Philly Family Court Building, with the marble columns, the 30-minute security check-in, and the grand holding pen for families, workers, and hungover child advocates. We'd all take turns on the wall charger, sitting on the dirty squeaking floors. The children, dancing, crying, running back and forth, screaming—their voices used to bounce across all that stone, reverberating up into the high roof while we all waited for our cases to get called.

Ten years ago, the city built a new Family Court. It's all glass and looks like an airport, and families don't crowd in through its doors and wait in a giant room like cattle or chattel anymore. There are televisions now that stream PBSKids for the children to watch. The waiting hasn't changed. I have known this child for four years out of the seven that he has been on this earth.

In his fifth year, he made his first court appearance alongside me, and I watched him sink into the inexplicable waiting that comes with court time—a unique temporal experience I once thought myself to be accustomed to, and seasoned in as a product of the many machines that whirr on for this country's poorest, most inconvenient families, youth, and individuals.

This was not this child's first experience with waiting, whether for visitation, or for the city-wide daycare subsidy to come through, or for a COVID-lockdown to expire. It was not his first experience with the chaotic and unpredictable machinations of adult relationships, and the hard truths of foster care, racialized care, disability, class, generational trauma, a global pandemic. When he first came to me at three years old, he only had a few words, and I went frantic with setting up evaluations, medical appointments, childcare, and wrap-around services. And the machine reminded us both to wait. There can be no urgency in the care of a Black child. Prevention and proactivity are privileges reserved for other children.

We had to wait for the paperwork to come in with all the insurance cards and eligibility verifications, and we waited with each other, like, "Well, I guess we gotta wait til we know each other now too." And while we waited for the machine, we got on with that impossible work of care and domesticity, impossible to do in such liminal temporalities as those that come with being case-managed and court-ordered. Sitting next to him in Family Court, watching his feet kick, and hearing his fruitless questions of *Are we done yet? Can we go home?*, I become aware of another five year old I know, who sits on the other side of me, invisible to most, but the child looks just like me and shares my name. By five years old, 2700 miles away in Los Angeles County, California, I had already sat through institutional time. Throughout preschool and kindergarten, I haunted the waiting rooms of lockdown juvenile behavioral health institutions where my older brother was held. I endured my brother's lengthy evaluations by eating the good hospital cookies, drinking the hot chocolate, and generally fawning at the frontline and administrative staff, who marveled at how I could occupy myself for the four hours needed to complete these assessments. But as I entered kindergarten, my brother managed to enter a free fall deeper into the maturing—and increasingly lucrative—juvenile detention system. In the 1990s, juvenile detention facilities in Southern California were bursting with children, especially Black and brown boys, and from 1990 to the early 2000s, juvenile facilities, boot camps, and other institutions meant to habilitate wayward adolescents having the highest populations in history, with Los

Padrinos juvenile detention center holding over 700 youth in 1990 when it was originally built to house 400 (Jovenes[cr1] Inc., 2023).

At five or six years old, I experienced my first juvenile criminal court hearing at the one-stop shop of juvenile detention proceedings, Los Padrinos Juvenile Hall, defunct as of 2019. I sat rigid next to my father while the attendees were read out loud. I remained still so that I could be invisible and continue being allowed to witness, be present, and attached to my father, who had no childcare that day, and so brought me to his only remaining minor son's criminal hearing.

I had fallen asleep to *Night Court* and *Judge Judy*. The court room wasn't unfamiliar, but I remember being shuffled into a wood-paneled room, not unlike church or some sort of auditorium, dissociating through the drone of grownup pomp and circumstance. The carpets I remember are still covered with dust, but I may be misremembering.

There's a memory of our shoes squeaking on the shiny floors—I may be mixing this up with the marble of the old Philly Family Court, or maybe the disinfected terrazzo in the art deco lobbies of one of the psychiatric hospitals that held and fed my mother for weeks and months at a time, while my father and me waited at home. Or maybe the polished concrete of the community clinic where my dad and I stood in line for hours waiting with dozens of other Californians for low-cost antibiotics, or a free round of childhood immunizations.

Now I am 35 again, and a week after the family court hearing, I'm back on the auction block shuffling into the overflow room where we can witness my friend's sentencing remotely, from another courtroom one floor below in a federal courtroom off Market Street. Unlike Juanita Kidd Stout Municipal Courthouse, which was often populated with jurors and defendants and generally a microcosm of Philly in and out of elevators and mediation rooms, this courthouse was empty, immaculate, and militaristic in its formalities and access.

There are so many of us here; for him, we had to wait in another room. I struggle to connect with the others here—so many who haven't seen each other in a long time. They all hold each other and seem so rooted together, consoling one another in these spaces. I have never seen such a spectacle of love in a place like a courthouse before this.

And I can't touch any of it, or they me, because as fat wet snow flakes slap the pavement in Old City Philadelphia 2023, it's also 1996, and 89 degrees. I'm eight years old, sitting outside Los Padrinos juvenile detention center on a hot glittering sidewalk, with 20 other unsupervised children, made to wait outside the doors while our parents visited our institutionalized siblings.

And I keep on reading my Stephen King book when one of them, a 15 year old or something, stands over me and says, "You can't read, you're not really reading that!" I keep a leg cocked ready to kick this kid in the knees if he gets any closer. The sun is still high. It'll probably be another two hours out here, but at least the book is long. I'm also eight years old and waiting in the lobby of the psychiatric hospital, playing "Hot cross buns" and "oh my darling clementine" on the piano they have set up in there, while I imagine my mother thrashing in a hospital bed, tied down by restraints. And I imagine my wooden father at her bedside, with nothing much to say except maybe a prayer. Or he may sit in a corner of her room while she stares blankly. Or maybe this time Dr. Ferguson joined him in her room, or met him in the hall. But all of this is a black box, an extension of my waiting mind. I used to wait at windowsills of different bedrooms in different apartments for many existential voids and possibilities. Brothers who will never come home, or who will only set upon one of these many apartments on the way to age 17, when I got here to Philadelphia. Eight moves, seven of which were in North Long Beach, Paramount, Norwalk, and Bellflower California. One of which was across the country.

I'm still waiting, on my most afflicted nights, for all my disappeared to reappear. Some did or do, and don't.

I'm waiting. There's a recess and the judge let all 150 of us out. I'm waiting in a cafe around the corner. I'm waiting in the security line, waiting in the blowing snow. And then outside the courtroom, and then in the elevator. I wait for my rideshare back West and catch a trolley to where my kid waits for me in his after school program.

I remember all the crimes my friends and I have endured in isolation. We all stopped waiting for a day in court; we stopped waiting early because of parentification and chronic disappointment. Justice doesn't come in a courtroom. Only heartbreak and invisibility.

For me, the temporal experience of interfacing with institutions as a Black person is one that has been lifelong, chronic, and repetitive. I have become a champion of inexplicable waiting, for a warehouse worker to pick up the phone, for healthcare, for so-called "justice," for emergency services to show up. It has been absurd and surreal to live the physical and emotional expectations put on me as a Black person who has been subjected to these machinations. It has been absurd and surreal to grow up masking the effects of these expectations on me, so as to move through the American Public School system and into the American Workforce [tm**]**.

Mad Black futurisms: Toward a Black time cure for ancestral wounds

Zimbardo's Time Perspective Theory (Zimbardo et al., 2012) places human experience temporally, with distinct dynamics associated with the past, present, and future. For people living with Complex Post-Traumatic Stress Disorder (C-PTSD), those distinct experiences of time become less salient, and more collapsed. There is a quantum nature to the lived experience of PTSD, especially the sort that is pervasive, historical, and never-ending. "There is not post-," and, even worse, the tool of culture is distorted into a survival mechanism.

C-PTSD in the context of massive historical or cultural trauma, like the ones Black people in America continue to face today, creates a particular challenge to the idea of "healing." To access employment, income, food, and relationships, Black people must move deftly in a mainstream, capitalist, white temporalities that value wellness, youth, ability, and productivity over all (Philips, R., 2025; Philips, R., 2022; McCartney, R., & Belknap, T. (2017); Philips, R. (2020). At the same time, Black people must operate under the scrutiny of such a system, as well the real temporalities and ghosts of institutionalization, incarceration, and racialized surveillance. Such a massive wound requires radical re-imaginings of Black trauma, Black mental health, and ancestral healing.

In 2017, I ran a workshop in North Philly called "Remember the Future" where we weighed these different time spaces and its relationship to our experiences in the neighborhood surrounding The Village of Arts and Humanities, where the workshop occurred.

This intergenerational group of neighbor-artists met weekly in the dead of winter to explore Time Travel and Memory as a healing practice. I thought that communicating about "trauma" could better be done with local conceptions of time, healing, and memory—ones that were distinctly spiritual, art/creativity based, and ones that were based on local wisdom, elders, intergenerationality, etc.

The model around psychoeducation regarding trauma at the agency was that we needed to redefine "trauma" in some way that was more "understandable" to our local population. I argued at meetings that we did not need to find a way to explain trauma to Philadelphians, but rather find a fruitful, useful space and practice for people to plug into so that the language came naturally, and learning came out of relationship to others in their community.

But engaging neighbors in a "writing workshop" exploring time travel and memory as a way to heal neighborhood trauma was an easy entree into what became a deep exploration of how trauma has affected our ability to be flexible temporally, and to avoid "stuckness" in any one temporal state.

This workshop formed a foundation of success that I have carried with me into Deep Space Mind 215's work since we began in earnest in 2021.

While my bosses from the agency that sponsored my work didn't attend the final reading and art show where our participants shared their writing on trauma with their community, I committed to my memory the feelings of authenticity and effectiveness—of a success defined by participants and facilitators rather than the institutions that search for grant outcomes in exchange for capital. The participants of that writing workshop felt heard, were able to share and express personal and neighborhood histories. They were able to connect in dialogue across generations and were able to visibly accommodate each other's madnesses, neurodiversities, and physical disabilities to ensure equitable participation. Most importantly, because the group was created by people with shared lived experience of institutionalization and community violence, the buy-in from neighbors was deeply impactful and led to a winter season full of rich conversation and connection.

Western therapeutic practice cannot on its own address the massive control that institutions, the state, and police have over the everyday lives of Black people, and others who mainstream mental health care is inaccessible and ineffective.

In Philadelphia, it will take more than talk therapy to address the immense powerlessness that many of us facing mental health challenges have felt in the face of the numerous racist machines that continue to grind up our neighbors.

I turn to Afrofuturism, disabled futures, the madness of "radical hope" (Hill-Jarrett, 2023), the creative power that comes with Black madtime (Bruce, 2021), and the hauntology that defines Black existentialism to work toward a more flexible, powerful framework of theory and practice to address C-PTSD, or Black Ancestral Trauma at both the individual and community level. This requires the work of building Life-Affirming Infrastructure, utilizing story circles, political education, and the practice of tapping into the madness of the Black radical imagination to conjure new realities of care (Page & Woodland, 2023).

Afrofuturism and its creative applications back at the Village of Arts and Humanities were a handy, locally based tool to deliver this workshop and others similar to it, and I fundamentally rely on it as a mental health practice. Committing to a framework of centering Mad Black futurisms in service of healing deep seated, ancestral, racialized trauma and beyond that can open us up to the possibility of collective liberation work.

We were able to put into practice and dialogue elements of Zimbardo's *Time Cure,* like the Zimbardo Time Perspective Inventory, and his 5 Time Theory (Zimbardo, P., Sword, R., & Sword, R., 2012), while keeping in mind hyperlocal and ancestral practices group members brought into the space. Zimbardo's framework included accessible language that allowed participants to examine their own relationships to the past, present, and future, and to analyze those relationships for health and fluidity, as well as transcendence and coping strategies used to manage complex PTSD symptoms.

One divergence did remain, however, from Zimbardo's *Time Cure* as divorced from historical or communal experience. Being "stuck" in time for residents of North Philadelphia, while inconvenient, painful, and at times harmful for our neighbors, also represented a strong desire for history to not be forgotten.

Thankfully, our workshop was built by people with shared cultural experiences, and we were able to incorporate dialogue about cultural practices that overlap with Zimbardo's conceptions of time as it relates to trauma healing. Some of these discussions included Black spiritual practices like Candomblé, Hoodoo, Black Catholicism, while others included Black communal traditions like storytelling by elders, and still others from youth-built practices like rap and spoken word. Together we explored our own time balances and discussed barriers to a balanced, healthful temporality—one that values the lessons of the past, acknowledges present need, and works toward a hopeful future.

#

Time travel: Honoring the Black temporality

The earliest iterations of Deep Space Mind and related workshops like "Remember the Future" committed participants and facilitation to the idea that all psychic states, at least while in the communal space, would be honored and valued as legitimate human experience that deserved witnessing, validation, and attention.

From the perspective of dealing with massive trauma, and the resulting C-PTSD, this means finding value in the flashbacks, steps backwards, the scramble to be present and survive, holding on by our nails to this reality. Of honoring our dreams, hopes, and beliefs, even when they are negative or rooted in hurt.

In *How to Go Mad without Losing Your Mind,* La Marr Jurelle Bruce defines "madtime" in the context of intersecting alternative temporalities of black time, queer time, and crip time, and in opposition to Western Standard Time, a temporality birthed in capitalism and racialized labor (Bruce, 2021). Madtime allows for the joyfulness of imagination and divinity of creativity of Black people, like the manic temporalities of Nina Simone, which drove her to become a forceful voice for Civil Rights during her career.

For Black people, acknowledging these fluid temporalities, the vividness of our nostalgia, the connectedness of our songs, our shared anxieties, and the synchronicities in our stories as survivors of the trans-Atlantic slave trade is a form of storytelling and witnessing that is integral to the Black Time Cure. And this storytelling and witnessing are communal and cultural. In the Philadelphia context, I have seen this be most effective when the storytelling and witnessing result in practical, lived improvements to the real environment, whether it's through a new resource for the neighborhood or a collective piece of art that can be viewed by the public. Interventions meant to heal ancestral trauma, especially in our local context, must acknowledge and interact with these temporal realities, particularly because structural racism directly targets Black people's time and temporal stability.

Whether it's through incarceration—systems involvement among children and youth, underpayment, and overwork—white culture interacts with Black communities often through the theft of time, especially time shared with other Black people. In Philadelphia, school closures, as one example, have robbed newer generations of neighborhood identity and loyalty and shared memories of proms and car washes—memories that older generations of Philadelphians cherish. This cultural rift between elders and young people further drives disconnection, a lack of storytelling and history sharing, and perpetuates the collective isolation residents feel under the pressure of gentrification, displacement, and disenfranchisement.

Acknowledging the fluidity of Black temporality, however, also venerates the ability of the Black collective to make and remake futures together. The pandemic and coinciding uprisings for Black lives across the country made very clear how much more proactive and powerful on-the-ground neighborhood cohesion and visioning can be, especially when compared to the dangerously slow mechanisms of traditional carceral systems of care, like the local homelessness service system or mental health care system. With the uprisings sprung up an energy and appetite for new systems, radical hope, and innovation.

And it's within that wave that Deep Space Mind 215 found its footing, in service of the mad Black belief that we will be here, and we will make this reality livable and joyful for all of us.

#

Manic Pixie nightmare - Mel Brown

At times I wonder about my utility in what appears to me as late-stage capitalism here in the West. I daily question if we are in the last years of the human epoch on earth. I live in the Western colony of the United States of America, notably known as Turtle Island of the Indigenous according to their spacetime. Today, my struggle is to survive a surveillance state that punishes Black people for being Black, creates barriers for higher economical class climb while monetizing off of sickness via the medical industrial complex, coupled with a field of care work that thrives on surplus people (Cutlass et al., 2016). This multi-pronged crisis is the legacy of mental health work both as consumers and providers of care. It is observed through generations of family members who were infirmary nurses, by the bedside of families with loved ones in underfunded state hospitals of their time, and the many of now ancestors who've lost their battle to addiction and homelessness for generations. Who are all these surplus people? They are considered as a class of people who are frontline, low-waged workers, depending on their credentials, of course, that the elite class capitalize from the labor and bodies of unfairly paid and overworked. Some of these people are more informal caretakers, disabled folks, and most importantly people who are detained in the carceral injustice system (Cutlass et al., 2016). Navigating the mental health industrial complex as a neurodivergent multi-diagnosed young mother, and low-waged healthcare worker, forced me into early adulthood. Quickly after being system involved, I experienced the passive violence of individuals at agencies. I distinctly remember the disdain of the workers at social service agencies who gatekept resources and faithfully clocked out of their desk jobs, pleased with themselves. Although surplus people themselves, these agents are not one of us even though many of them looked like us. Internalized anti-Blackness is not realizing how they uphold institutions that penalize Black poor mothers for their lack of better choices, in the name of social services.

Today, I belong to the fleet of Black femmes who are educated, credentialed, over-qualified, and in hundreds of thousands of dollars in financial debt to higher educational institutions, that begged us to attend for their numbers. The combination of my first-hand experience and on-the-ground practice in care work that spans over a decade in the city of Philadelphia makes me equipped to have both a perspective as a service provider and, more importantly, as a consumer. I cannot say that I know what's left to my community during what feels like you're in the seat of a falling global empire. The American empire provides the matches and bullets to a world that is perpetually on fire and at war. Survival is impossible without community. Can our stories suffice as a cumulative knowledge for survival? Yes, when our individual stories paired with an archival praxis, surplus people have a duty to do more than just survive in the seat of a burning empire. We must thrive and pass on our experiences to future generations. What happened to me is not isolated; instead, I offer that what happened to me was and is just a ripple in a vast ocean of similar afflictions and happenings.

In 2002, I was hospitalized for the first time and released after spending a week in the Saint Louis University Hospital psych ward. I am eighteen, barely sober, with fire-engine-red dreadlocks. When I was released from the hospital with my pink long johns and some popular band t-shirt, I walked out. Eager for release and without shoes, I crossed the street and made a phone call to a friend asking for a ride home. I am there, riding in the car with peers who have fallen off the wagon. Since the age of 16,

I've been in a rehabilitation program for substance abuse where I found myself hugging strangers casually saying, "I love you" to my white suburban peers who were described as troubled teens. I'd just graduated from the infamous sobriety cult program located in the midwest and landed myself in Alcoholics Anonymous with others who also graduated from the sobriety program. I'd dropped out of my former high school to receive treatment and now, after graduating from the sobriety program, I'm released into the world as a recovering teen not knowing what to do next. I begged for my feelings of not belonging and grief to be over. Later that summer, I ran away and returned pregnant.

I can never be here fully. Chronic slow-released trauma jolts my brain, and my memory slips, leaving behind gaps. I made myself transform the social rejection of being a surplus person fuel to flame my ambitions. As I burned out, I realized, what I thought was propelling my ambitions of class climbing cost me something greater. Growing up in a single-parent middle-class household run by a matriarch who centered on men and the Black church left me as the only female child, to challenge religious dogma around gendered servitude, mental illness, and poverty shame leaving behind yet another metastasized site of social rejection to be healed. I never felt that my life had any inherent value outside of providing care to my family and community. It took me years to unlearn the myth of meritocracy, Black excellence, and Black cultural belief systems that centered one's value on how success-fully one could assimilate into the status quo or dominate class through means of social climbing. I was Sysiphus, at the bottom of the hill contemplating life and death while pushing my invisible mental illness up it to, nowhere. To the viewer, I am a champion, capable, my high functioning mask afforded me to neglect the limitedness of my humanity and basic needs. Perfectionism eventually corroded my brain, with self criticism, hypervigilance, all products of what I consider today as Black excellence trauma.

Poem:
a walking disaster
left side of my mouth between tooth
    (blank) and tooth (blank) there's a gap
I have a scar on my left knee from
    running away from a boy who choked
    me for the first time
with your main character energy
and the unceasing inner-narrator who
    sounds like Billy Zane from the movie
    Demon Night
your jaw is askew
and you walk funny
your voice too low
it only mattered if you were beautiful
let them meet all of your people

\#

A social worker's history of running - Rashni Stanford

\#

Alondra Boulevard

Some of my earliest memories were in Long Beach, California, where I remember using the black plastic fist of an afro pick as a teether while a neighbor braided my hair for my tired mother, who worked something scary called "the graveyard shift" at the airport. Or watching WWF Saturday mornings with my brothers as they argued over their favorite wrestlers and practiced suplexes on me. I noted the occasional break-ins, or the fights my brothers would have with my parents, but otherwise lived in the bliss of a young child growing up on the block.

I saw footage of the Rodney King riots at the age of four on our television in the living room, and if I stretch my brain enough, I may even recall some concern that my brothers were missing in that moment. And suddenly, the narrative in my memories jumps forward some, to when we have a Nintendo system, and we all play Super Mario Bros. together on my brothers' bunk bed. My mom is there too, and she speed runs through levels effortlessly when she's awake, and I believe my family, my two older brothers, my old dad, my mom, and me are pretty special.

I don't realize though that these spoils my brothers made off with were just some of the baggage the riots would spark in our family. Police presence in Long Beach became more intense, and landlords became shadier in how they distributed housing. We left Long Beach, the story went, because of the trouble my brothers were getting into, and the lack of stability in our lease. My brothers spent a lot of time dodging community violence, avoiding school, and running the streets. Our landlord didn't really want to deal with Black people any more, it seemed, especially not any "out of control boys" running around with stolen goods.

I moved three times by the age of six, each time progressively further away from Long Beach, and all in the direct aftermath of the Rodney King riots. With every move, it seemed family members peeled off one by one.

Inevitably our escape route from Long Beach ran along Alondra Boulevard, the thoroughfare that leads you from Gardena, and all the Gateway Cities of Los Angeles County to Buena Park in Orange County. Ironically Alondra Boulevard's existence is said to be a memorial to the racist land grab (Evains, 2022).

First, we moved to Paramount, just a mile or two away and butt-up to Compton, to a low-income rental occupied primarily by Spanish speakers, and then up the street to a larger apartment complex that was Black owned and occupied. Then, after the shooting death of my oldest brother, we moved farther out to suburban city of Norwalk, which still had its share of gangs and apartment complexes with their own stories of misery and anguish.

Or maybe it was my family that brought the misery to Belshire Blvd. We tried our best to outrun the riots, my brothers' institutionalizations, the death of my siblings, one to gun violence, and one sister before I could properly meet her died during childbirth, leaving behind two children.

But even in the townhouse complex in Norwalk, all that my family ran from came creeping back, especially when no attention had been paid to my brother's murder, my mother's increasing mental illness, and my remaining older brother's unchecked trauma and resulting behavioral issues that saw him frequently removed from our household and community.

When we first moved into the complex of townhouses, the six-year-old me thought, "Wow a real upstairs-downstairs house!" and I hoped for some forever-ness here, superstitiously hoping things would pan out here the way they did in two story homes in TV sitcoms.

The complex was full of Black and Korean kids, and for a time, we were free to wander within the gates of the complex, which offered mundane adventures like stealing back one of our bikes from the backyard of a neighboring house, or picking guava fruit from an overhanging tree branch with the help of boost from a friend. Or learning to Double Dutch, playing hide and seek, or handball against someone's garage. The attached units all had their rear garages facing the shared driveway, shuttered with an automated green painted iron gate that was supposed to bounce back open if a child or bike was detected, but didn't always.

We played street hockey on rollerblades down that center drive, practiced the butterfly to TLC songs, sang the Free Willy theme song at each other's birthday parties. We played Barbies meets X-men and lounged in our garage building endless Lego complexes and neighborhoods.

It was the mid-1990s, and the rent was $800 for a bi-level two bedroom townhome with a washing machine and garage. This was stretching the upper limit of my parents' shared income. My father was a retiree of a large airline company where he had worked cleaning and prepping planes before boarding. My mother at the time we moved in was a food handler at the same company back when they served the whole plane full meals for free. Most of our family friends were workers at LAX, and I enjoyed endless crime and romance novels collected from planes at the end of a flight and set aside for when my father and I came over to visit and catch up.

It wasn't long before the idyllic life we tried to settle into became upended by the ghosts of Long Beach, although now that I am older, I realize our family wasn't the only one whose hood problems followed us around Southern California. My brother, at 14 years old had linked up with some other troubled teenagers and quickly began running away again, returning only in one or two-day spurts to set up a Sega Genesis he had pilfered so he could teach me a fatality or two, or to grab some clothes or drop off some fish he had caught in the LA river.

In those spurts, he would regale me with tales of close encounters with police, mall security guards, and his friends from the old neighborhood, who had all been scattered in institutions, group homes, and foster families throughout the area.

While entertained, I sensed a darkness moving over all of us. Interactions with other children became darkened as my brother started fights, and he and his friends brought police presence to the apartment building. Soon, our family became one to be avoided, and when I roamed the gated complex, I did it alone. My brother and mother were dangerous, and I imagined myself while I played alone, a portal into the psych hospitals and supervised detention programs they inhabited. When the parents of my friends ignored my knocks, I agreed with them internally— *It's for the best, I'd just drag your children down, my family is known for this.*

When my brother ran away for the last time, he was apprehended and placed in juvenile detention, separating me from him for six or so years. While my brother's fate was worked out in juvenile court, my mother had her first in a long series of psychotic episodes leading to stints of institutionalization that lasted a month to four months at a time. I spent a lot of time during the length of elementary school in psychiatric hospital waiting rooms, family therapy rooms, touring residential treatment centers for my brother, and attending his often graphic court hearings, where my presence as a first or second grader was often forgotten.

I understood why my brother wanted to run, but I also saw how heavy his price was for doing so. And I thought he was foolish for not being patient, for not waiting for an opportunity or a road, rather than barreling his way out the way he did. *Why make it so much harder*, I would think. Kids were getting shot left and right, especially back in Paramount and Long Beach, where our roller-coaster seemed to start, and half of the teenagers I knew were in a group home or bootcamp somewhere. Inside our house was terrifying, but the threat of getting jumped, killed, arrested, or otherwise institutionalized concerned me more.

My father and I became very close at this time, as we were left alone together in the house, and did a lot of ad hoc troubleshooting around my mother when she was home—we attempted to keep her calm on our own so that EMTs or police would not have to be called. When we were unsuccessful, we often planned to stay out playing tennis until late in the night, hoping she would be asleep when we returned. Often we would sleep in the garage, or on the sidewalk near the tennis courts at the park in Cerritos, to avoid her pacing, ranting, and violent threats. When she was feeling low, and weepy, I would be tasked with keeping her company while my father bought some groceries or alleviated tensions with the property manager.

When my mother was inpatient, life was easygoing and peaceful, and all that teamwork in crisis led to collaboration around the house, and mutual peacekeeping. We became addicted to a simple routine, school, drive through, library, the park, home for *The Simpsons* and maybe an episode of *20/20*, and then we retreated to our rooms and fell asleep to some books. Or Jerry Springer in my case. In those quiet times at the park, I was able to relentlessly question my father on his life, and what led us to where we were then.

My father would tell me how he himself ran away from his native Guyana when he was 14, how he skipped school most of the days because he couldn't fall in line enough to avoid getting beaten by the Anglican teachers. He avoided his mother and her beatings at home, and spent his days in the cane fields, or on the black beaches near his home eating raw shrimp whole. The story goes that he hopped onto a ship as a young teen and became a sailor sometime in the 1930s, until he found his way to Ellis Island as a young man in 1942 before joining the U.S. Merchant Marines as a cook and serving in the Korean War.

Even back then I realized the parallels between my brothers and my father—running from the callousness of a Black mother, a colonial education system, and a world not built for young Black boys without a family to protect them.

At the same time, I saw the shortcoming of my father's narrow-minded idea that his ancient version of Caribbean-style parenting would hold up in working-class Black Southern California, reeling from youth violence, mass incarceration, and a new brand of family institutionalization.

My father had no clue how to handle child rearing crises, domestic violence, or severe mental illness without inviting an institution into his home. He was desensitized to the institutional machine because he had been adopted by the U.S. military industrial complex, and there was no G.I. bill for him, so he had no economic standing as a reward.

He had no idea that calling the police once on a wayward child in 1990 would enroll the entire family into truancy surveillance, welfare checks, group homes, residentials, and eventually the court house.

My brother consistently ran back to the homes of friends who understood him and protected him in the street, and my father never saw these families as resources or supports. My father consistently called the cops on all of us: my mother when she was violent, my brother when he was missing, and myself on days when the 1st grade seemed too unbearable to sit through, and I holed up in my bedroom with daytime television.

The three of us—my mother, father, and I—fell into a delicate dance of muddled familial roles. My father and I filled in the gaps for the missing family members and their fluctuating capacities. I let my dad know when my mom was on the phone cursing out her boss at the airlines. I was the first to know she lost her promise of pension with that job at the age of seven years old. I became preoccupied with maintaining our security deposit when she began pouring bleach and powdered detergent on the carpets, causing strange, hardened stains up and down the staircase. I had come to see as a symbol of failed stability. My mother revolved in and out of psychiatric inpatient stays. I split her caretaking duties with my father, who spent his time bumbling through interactions with social workers, child welfare and juvenile court staff, behavioral health workers and psychiatrists.

I also split the job of looking after myself with my parents. From the late age of six to ten years old, I found ways to stay out of the way while my dad was preoccupied with the logistics of caring for my mother. I read voraciously and watched late night TV into the morning so that I could sleepwalk as peacefully as possible through the school day. I wore a veneer of normalcy at school and church to protect our household from more institutional involvement. Even when my mother, in the throes of an episode, would call child welfare on my father, I would stun the social workers with my academic achievements and calm conversation.

I wandered the complex alone probably for a year or so before running into one of my first sexual abusers, the father of a playmate. Perhaps when we kids played together more, he had access to me. But in those dark times between seven and ten years old, when the house was shaken up by institutionalization, I found myself in his townhome a lot, after school or on weekends when being out of the house seemed like the easiest way to stay out of the cross fire, and to keep from being an added calculation to my dad's caretaking agenda.

While my six-year-old self found it hard to hide behavioral signs that I was being sexually abused, I learned quickly that sexual behavior taught to me elsewhere was not welcome in most company, and so those experiences had to be well hidden until new perpetrators made themselves known to me.

After three or four of my mother's episodes and subsequent hos-pitalizations, my brother's removal from our home, the pariah status I had internalized, and the growing frequency of sexual violence I began inexplicably experiencing, I started to agree with my brother in his absence.

If I wanted a life of my own, I would need to run at some point, and so I began by running into dreams, fantasies, stories I made up about my future self. I found times when I could be still with myself the most comforting, even when I was consumed by night-marish, self-loathing thoughts, it felt like running. I could separate from my body for hours and hours at a time, no TV required.

Upon turning eight, I decided to walk out of the side gate of the complex and explore the enclave surrounding our block on my own. I'd walk to Stater Brothers and steal beef jerky, or hover around the donut shop during the school day to see who recognized me, or who would stop and ask why I wasn't in school. No one ever did.

I considered myself much more sensible and patient in my run-ning than my brother. I would gather information before I left; I would look for the right opportunity instead of throwing myself into the streets.

At the library, I searched for books on throwaway kids and miss-ing persons, scoured the YA section for stories of kids who got away and got to be free from institutions like family and residen-tial treatment, and who thrived in spite of their parents' lack of caring capacity.

By the time I was ten, I had gone through countless involuntary commitments with my mother, calling plays with frontline emer-gency workers in one apartment or another to safely get her into an ambulance. I was desensitized to anything that wasn't a promise of leaving the destroyed apartments I seemed fated to inhabit. I was becoming desperately depressed and would often spend multiple days in a row unmoving in my bed, unable to rejoin the waking world with my full embodiment.

I watched my father's age showing, and my mother's mental health becoming dangerous and unbearable. I hadn't seen my brother in years—my father seemed unable to keep up with the visits and team meetings that the residential treatment center was requesting of him. We had left a security deposit in Norwalk and ran to yet another apartment complex, this time in the working-class city of Bellflower, California. I began to wonder if we wouldn't all die together the way families did in the true crime I began to consume from 20/20 specials, and late night TV like Dateline and Profiler.

At that time, I had gotten my hands on a series of novels from the 1970s and 1980s written by the Catholic-founded youth shelter, Covenant House. The titles of these novels were vintage trendy names of teen girls and at least one boy, ones like "Lori" or "Terri" or "Debbi." Each of these were propagandized case studies of young adults who ran away and found themselves on the streets, and who lived hard before finding Covenant House, where they got cleaned up and built new lives for themselves. I was aware these books were fictionalized advertisements, but I studied them anyway for tactics, strategies, and shared truths about growing up and coming of age alone, without the support of a family.

There was an unspoken silence my father and I shared about what went on inside my home, and it meant family friends who occasionally let me stay with them during my mother's worst nights, regarded me with restrained care. No one knew what to say about my mother's hospitalizations, or the rumors of the behaviors and scenes that she was a part of. No one knew how to appropriately address my brother's delinquency, his absence, and no one spoke of my dead brother, and any of the pains that drove him as a 17 year old into the street in the first place, where he would be unprotected from gunfire.

And in that way, no one spoke of me or any of the madnesses I endured as a Black girl child, or on land me and my brother have come to know as haunted with the ghosts of all the displaced, houseless, thrown away, and institutionalized. Growing up on occupied Tongva land, Los Angeles County was saturated with the color of housing scarcity, rents constantly climbing, fleeing gun violence here and there, property managers always changing out, neighbors and old friends scattered everywhere after the riots—Whittier, Norwalk, Lakewood, The Inland Empire, Ontario, Pomona.

It seemed the benign neglect employed by officials and cops during the Rodney King uprisings had done its intended job and created a normalcy of displacement for Southern California's working-class Black families.

Home seemed to be a series of leases, and dependent on one's perceived emotional stability while inhabiting Blackness. One could not at once be housed, be Black, and be visibly mad. And so, for me, it seemed I could not be home, or should not be so foolish to believe there was one for me somewhere while I remained attached to my family's madness.

Still, during my mother's last hospital stay in California, when my father let me know that we were moving again, I felt enough hope to sift through a *For Rent* magazine and have a hand in our next place. I circled properties within our budget, not too far away so that my middle school placement would be in jeopardy. I thought I would try one more year in my father's house if we found an apartment with some other kids there, some normalcy, less silence, and maybe some respite from my mother's violent episodes.

With my mother in the hospital this last time, I found my mind filled with plots to run away and disappear into the streets of Los Angeles County. Sometimes I dreamt hopeful, feeling equipped to beat the odds—I wouldn't end up on skid row, I would be strategic. Other times, I found myself obsessing over the ways child victims of murder, like JonBenet Ramsay, were able to have their cases poured over, turned over by millions of people on Fox during TV specials. I read news about disappearing youth, and trafficking victims, and I felt self-destructive, pulled perhaps by what I felt was an inevitable fate. In this way, I began to understand the way my brother crashed out even more.

I found myself completely disconnected at school, unable to retain much information or complete projects. I stole spare moments to put my head down and dream, about finding an adult willing to take me in, of approaching my parents' old friends, or propositioning day laborers to harbor me in exchange for sexual favors.

One day, my father drove me after school to one of the apartment complexes I had circled, one called Sierra Gardens. We quickly toured the drab 2 bedroom, which seemed suitable, even without including a refrigerator. While my dad spoke to the property manager, I did a quick lap around the property, searching for other kids, for Black families, or any sense of connection I could look forward to.

Sure enough, I ran into gangs of children throughout the complex. They asked, "You moving in here?" I huffed an affirmative, "I think so!" before returning to the manager's office. This would be something worth waiting around for, I thought.

#

Sierra Gardens

I ended up spending my middle school years and half of high school at the Sierra Gardens, an apartment building serving low- and middle-income Black and brown families on the Bellflower/Paramount city line. It became the longest home I inhabited in California, and it gave me some vital clues as to what to search for in the way of home, community, and connection as an adult. It's a blessing my father listened to me when I forced this decision, and I think of an example of a time when I had a distinct child's wisdom that needed to be trusted.

My mother lived with her sisters on the East Coast, where I safely visited her and the rest of my maternal family in Newark, Brooklyn, and Delaware.

This complex boasted three separate buildings, a toxic swimming pool serviced once a year with 2 tons of chlorine, and a semi-revolving community of what seemed like hundreds of kids and families throughout the years.

We celebrated birthdays, convinced each other's adults to watch us in the pool, played hide and seek until the stars came out, and went on long bike rides and walks to the local park, or the super-market for pickles or Hot Cheetos.

We would have sleepovers, make dinner, play endless games of Mancala, do each other's hair. My friends' parents and caregivers were loving and generous, and they raised me through some of my tenderest moments with bowls of gumbo, free sets of Alicia Keys' braids, and when my father's health declined, they provided me words of love and wisdom where my household—now filled with his hospital bed and my stepmother's homophobic disdain for me—had none.

The AOL installation disks got mailed out our way when I was 11, and the new internet provided respite from when the old things tried creeping into this reality, where I had friends, and where we were all survivors of violence, addiction, poverty, racism in one way or another. I catfished older men, played video games, and consumed endless amounts of media and information—another attempt to outrun the memories I still carried with me from the old apartments.

At the end of eighth grade, my father had his first in a long series of strokes that left him debilitated. My brother, now a young adult aged out of state care, returned home to look after my dad, and also to butt heads with my abusive stepmother, a CNA back in Brooklyn where she housed her daughter's brood in a brown-stone that she paid for with my father's airline pension checks.

On the first day of high school, the World Trade Center collapsed in an attack, and our school teacher played the footage in our homeroom. My remedial algebra teacher Mr. Garcia quickly ran down the geopolitical history of Afghanistan, Iraq, and the Bush lineage, and warned us against disinformation we may hear over the next four years. I went home, and my best friend's mother said the same, while preoccupied by the news ticker on the 24-hour news channels that had become popular at that time. The Y2K idealism had come and gone, and the internet for teens was flooded with graphic imagery of war within a year.

By the start of high school, my father was incapable of caring for me, and the situation in my household became unbearable once more, as my emerging queerness was clocked by my step-mother, even in the absence of any evidence or action on my part. Obsessed with keeping my history of sexual abuse secret, I was convinced that my mistreatment had to do with prior vic-timization she somehow became privy to.

Sometime in ninth grade, I returned from a trip to visit my mother in Newark to a room with no bed frame and no dresser. My clothes began to smell after being piled onto the floor in trash bags, and the mattress on the floor I slept on was full of bed bugs.

By the beginning of sophomore year of high school, I found our apartment door locked and was never allowed a key. I began staying at friend's houses until late in the night when I could sneak into the apartment's front window, or perhaps my brother would be sleeping on the living room couch and could let me in.

I became intensely depressed, back to the old comforts of cat-atonia, which sometimes lasted days. I became plagued at the same time with spells of sleep paralysis, nightmares, and muteness. I was selectively mute in eighth grade when my father first became ill, but in the depths of high school in California, this lasted much longer, and even my beloved friends in the complex could rarely rouse me, or get me to speak with them. I began enclosing myself in my own world inside my own mind space, where I could be left alone.

I was able to make it to school to play on the school's tennis team or to sing in the school musical with Drama Club. And for a time I was president of the community service club, where I had the eerie experience of handing out Christmas presents at the very apartment complex my brother was killed in front of. It had the same blue stucco, and for weeks after that, I walked around dissociated, with what seemed like cotton over my ears.

One night I came home from school and saw all my things packed into two plastic bags. I was being kicked out and had to go and live with my mother in Newark. And with that, I was running somewhere else, but this time alone.

#

Brick city and the path train

In Newark, my heart was broken for leaving Sierra Gardens, but my energy was renewed. It was a majority Black city that I had navigated since I was in elementary school. The Vailsburg neighborhood, Irvington shopping strip, and Penn Station were already cherished spaces in my memories, and the source of Caribbean treats like tamarind balls and ginger beer, and the East Coast fast fashions I would smuggle back in my luggage to reveal to my friends. I knew the way to the neighborhood park, and I knew the bus route that took me to Rainbow in Irvington, or to Broad and Market downtown.

And beyond Newark, I had memories of playing dominoes on a Bedstuy block with 100 family members and neighbors during my cousins kwe-kwe[1], and of taking the subway throughout the 1990s with my dad on the way to the ferry as a child.

There was still fear there, and pain there. During the summer and winter breaks I spent in the city with my mother, albeit under the supposed supervision of her older sisters, I experienced more sexual violence. Somehow on the opposite coast, my mother's needs continued to reduce the capacity of my alternative caregivers to look after me properly and to account for my safety. It always seemed that the two priorities were mutually exclusive: my safety versus my mother's mental stability. And now as a 15 year old, I was tasked with setting up my life on another coast, while caring for my mother, monitoring her behavior and her spending.

I had fears that my mother's mental state would reach the same extremes as those of my childhood and doubted my ability to manage them alone. However, when my aunts promptly moved down South when I arrived, there was little choice for me but to move forward.

In any case, the public transportation, my new humanities-centered magnet high school, and the jerk chicken patties being sold downtown invigorated me. Unlike the car-centered world I had come from, I could move freely with the help of school-issued bus tickets to get my needs met.

It felt like I got off the airplane, unpacked my black trash bags into the dining room that had been fashioned into my living space, and I got to work—finding a school to enroll in, then a job, and then maybe a couple of friends. I needed to get signed up for bus passes, and I needed to find the tennis coach. Mostly I needed to graduate and escape into adulthood in one piece.

Newark provided fertile ground for me to practice autonomous movement and network building all around the city. NJ Transit, the PATH train, and the MTA were my wings, and I could survey my new setting with so much more ease and grace.

I found two part-time jobs, one at the Newark Museum and one at a wing spot off market street. I found a group of fellow truant youth to skip school and buy bootleg NorthFace jackets in Chinatown, and to scheme on finding extra hours at the museum where we worked. The people in the city were friendly, direct, hilarious, and a million facets of Black. My West Indian classmates spoke so many different types of creole and patois, and my homies rooted in the South, or who had been in the New York area for generations, force-fed me crabs on the first of the month and placed Chinese food orders for me.

I had so much space to roam outside of the third-floor apartment I lived in with my mother. As she began to decline again, I spent more time outside, having adventures off the Christopher Street PATH Stop, or playing Dance Dance Revolution at the Newport Mall in Jersey City. I began organizing with other young people from Newark and NYC, participating in political education and anti-war movement work with local educators. I relished in the Black educators at University High School, and the teachers who poured into us beyond the classroom, gathering us politically with respect and care during the full-fledged War on Terror. We read *Invisible Man* and Howard Zinn, and I came to be grounded and confident in a city where its political history and place in resistance work were all around me. I learned about it from neighbors, teachers, students, wheatpastes, and community newspapers.

The senior year felt like a downhill descent toward the edge of a cliff alone. My father died in a nursing home that winter, and a few weeks before graduation, my mother suffered another major episode. During her institutionalization, I went through her paperwork to collect my social security card and birth certificate. I hadn't gotten into any of the colleges I applied to, and I had little familiarity with the details of going to college. Instead, I had focused on the prospect of housing, and a socially acceptable avenue to relocating far enough away to not remain my mother's ad hoc caregiver.

A few days after graduation, I got an email to apply to Drexel University's College of Media Arts and Design. I sent them a writing sample and application, got accepted, and got a ride from my cousin down to Philly for orientation.

Coming down 95, I saw the skyline rise over the horizon and felt disoriented because it looked so similar to Newark. I almost asked if we had somehow gotten turned around and ended up back in Jersey. Murals from the sides of buildings warmed my heart and reminded me of the murals back in California. Our exit was off 676, near Drexel, but I clocked Broad and Market from the highway, and a clear message in my head told me, "This is the place for you." The city felt inexplicably familiar, and any reluctance that rose in me was immediately dismissed. Something had called me to this place in my constant searching for an opportunity, an escape hatch. It had come in the form of a mass email to teens who had missed the FAFSA[2] deadline, and I was determined to make this run count.

Messages from personal history

Looking back, I see how I have been pulled into the ancestral spiral of displacement, community removal, and personal marronage as a last-ditch effort to make great change for myself. In the emptiness and uncertainty around "home" and rootedness that I felt growing up, I had inadvertently developed and uncovered ancestral strategies for living under the circumstances of running. I had inadvertently run into many examples of home and love, collecting them with me on my way out.

I had intended to come to Philadelphia to write horror movies about the apartments I grew up in, but I inevitably had to drop out in my second year over tuition fees and a lack of financial familial support.

Relying on my lived experiences in institutions, I entered the direct support professional pipeline, figuring that an entry-level social service job would be enough to pay rent and maybe secure health insurance, now that I was kicked out of the dorms. I worked at a crisis nursery up Germantown, where young children in crisis were cared for in a big gingerbread house by workers on shift. Most of the little ones had caregivers who had just gotten a new job and were still finagling child care, or their family's had moved to a shelter after a house fire and needed time to secure transportation to the child's original daycare. We had quaint regimens of shared meals, structured play and story-time, and lazy weekends taking long walks or languishing in the large backyard.

But there were times at that job where we were frontline emergency workers, accepting abused or neglected children under six years old directly from the blocks they were found on. I found myself glowing with pride and confidence in those moments. I saw how fearful and uncomfortable police officers were in handling children who wouldn't speak, how the cops lingered in the crisis nursery, as though they wanted to hang on to the one good thing they did that week. The feeling of providing a warm landing for a child who had been wandering the street in the middle of the night closed a circuit for me.

Like Britney Daniels, author of *Journal of a Black Queer Nurse*, the impossible work of humanizing care against the backdrop of violent systems invigorated me, and I began to pride myself in the brief but intense connection held with another human being in crisis (Daniels, 2023). And, like the Black neighbors who formed Freedom House and the first iteration of the modern paramedic profession, I was both a survivor and a frontline worker who hungered for innovation in care work (Hazzard, 2022)—in the care of Black families, Black children, and Black neighborhoods in crisis.

The work provided a rest from running. The city that provided me home told me loudly and clearly that I was to spend a good amount of time supporting the ones who have to run—whether from gun violence, family violence, gentrification and displacement, houselessness, and dissociation. I was told loudly and clearly—by way of numerous open houses posted on Monster.

com—that I must enter the residential treatment centers that raised my brother and all of his friends, and I had to see what I couldn't during our separation. And I realized all of those kids were runners too. In fact, a youth placement in a residential treatment center in Pennsylvania almost required the tendency to run away as an element of eligibility. A teen who ran was unfit for a community, and so, as a direct support professional, we made one together under the supervision of the institution.

It's almost 20 years now since I ran to this place, and I haven't had to leave yet, nor have I wanted to. I have found identity here as a youth worker with housing insecure teens and young adults. I have become a parent working in the foster system. I have worked in numerous shelters and organized alongside neighbors seeking stability in their neighborhoods and housing. I have made lifelong friends who help me raise my child, and they share with me their elders and their offspring to love on.

My roots have found shelter here, and I feel compelled to tend this ground so that all the Philadelphians who have raised and nurtured me have something steadier to stand on.

#

Black transplant lamentations - Rashni Stanford

#

After the 1980s, Black space nationally became fractured dimensionally, and so too did Black kinship bonds, rituals, spirituality, spiritual diversity, and creativity, as they all became reshuffled by shifts in education, class, migration, immigration, and an American culture desperate to erase the Black collective resistance of the past, and replace it with a reality where racism has been defeated. Those of us left behind were raised in conditions of isolation and broken care networks. The transmission of Black history and multigenerational settings necessary to provide rootedness, stability, and security in Black families and communities have been disrupted.

Philadelphia, in particular, a city entirely composed of strong, Black, tight-knit neighborhoods, has been hit with the ongoing legacy of benign neglect, homelessness, displacement, and gentrification. The effects on social bonds and mental health are tremendous and ever-present.

Just standing in line at a grocery store in the summertime, I could hear all of the "It's a damn shames" related to the lack of proper block parties and block party permits being offered by the city, or about shuttered pools and rec centers. Constant murmurings about programs and gatherings that should be ever-present, that every Black child should experience. My neighbors never allow the past to fade away—it is always in dialogue with the present, and it sets up a blueprint for action and future manifestation and repair.

Witnessing Philadelphia elders recount their own experiences of local history for the past few years has reminded me of all the collective memory Philadelphians walk with, from witnessing tanks and coping with clouds of tear gas on 52nd Street in 2020 to memories of the shock and horror of 1985's M.O.V.E bombing[3] smoke rising over the horizon. At the same time, unending violence abroad—in Haiti, Congo, Sudan, and Palestine—has me considering ancestral methods of memorial and collective grief and resistance in times of ongoing violence. The Abrahamic traditions that my ancestors found spirit inside of also call to me. As someone born in the seat of an empire that sends rockets in God's name, it feels right and true to wail and gnash. I feel we may not find our way back if we don't stop to do so before moving forward.

A Black psychiatrist from another deindustrialized city who sheltered me when I was young, Dr. Mindy Thompson Fullilove, wrote about the unique personal and collective trauma that comes with displacement and urban renewal in America's Black cities and neighborhoods. When traditional 3rd spaces in Newark, New Jersey, were erased by urban renewal, neighbors had to replace the lost ritual and connection that accompanied those community spaces, as well as maintain social networks in spite of the shifting landscape (Fullilove, 2016).

In the midst of massive shifts in the city, and in the repeated aftermath of weathering and rebuilding after crisis, it feels necessary to witness this hard work and to remember the losses as we move toward the future.

The city lament is an ancient narrative technology utilized throughout the Levant, Mediterranean, (Jacob, 2016) and arguably at times in the Black diaspora in the form of poetry and song. The years since 2020 and the bitter injustices that COVID-19 uncovered have weighed on me over the past four years. This city has minded and tended to me when I hit my own lows and experienced my own crises. I believe the city lament does some work to respect the spirit of this place that has held me, and can hopefully provide some deserved witnessing to the pain and growth that occurs here.

> *For Joshua Glenn of Youth Art & Self Empowerment project, Sul'Yah Williams, Jimmy Mao, Chynna Rogers, Dominique "Rem'mie" Fells, and the beloved gardeners of Pentridge Children's Garden. A portion of the following piece was a part of the 2024 Dreaming Deep Roots workshop, in collaboration with Word for Worlds Animation, Phillycam, and Philly Land Stewards.*

1.

My own children lost faith in me as they were ground into the mud of the land, their once beautiful rowhomes festering with wetness, mold, floods, melting in the heat, the raccoons take over their roofs and the squirrels their porches.

My own children live and die on soft porches in old age, repeating the same old stories of love and prosperity on the block. When the babies hear this, they believe it is an ancient myth, dubious but pleasant at times to listen to.

My children attend funerals of their elders, and their very young and their hearts are cold after so many lost. Bars and bureaucracy separate children from kin, in the mirror, they don't recognize each other, except in exchanges of paltry gifts, and shiny shoes made by the children of other countries with no other choice but to sew sew sew.

2.

Oh mother, you fed me like I was your own, and I wanna do right by you, so I will tell the truth.

We never knew your name; we only came for the low rents and the prestige of an institution to attach to. Forgive us trodding over you and all the bones of your children, for infiltrating every living wage and for the blinders of cash that keep us safe, warm, and sheltered.

We sucked up every studio apartment application, every leadership or entry-level, or middle manager position, every first-time home buyers' grant; we bought houses in the catchment areas that ensured the longest life expectancy for our seed.

We crossed the street at the sight of your children; we never spoke a word to the elders stewarding the crumbling homes we renovated around, and when the developers bought the grannies out, nobody blicks at our block parties.

This city's powerhouse of artistry stays passed over for celebrities, emphatic influencers, and gatekeepers called activists, organizers, and mavericks.

We made you an unfinished project. We ran when the tanks rolled through.

3.

Pouring libations, watching the lines blur between Gods, watching God appear before our eyes. In each other and the sun and the strength of the laughter of Philly's children. And watching those who claim to know this deity flap their mouths as they use the word to direct bombs back to everybody's Holy Land.

I didn't dream of the love of elders, but here it is suddenly and needed. It was in the seed I spirited away with me from the backdam where my mother played with my ghost as a child in a trench. Maybe she saw me there as a tadpole and whispered to me some blueprints for today. And maybe they called her mad back then, but I am still thankful.

Pouring libations at the beginning of a march for a dead Black girl, whose murderer I once knew, whose spirit makes us all more dangerous, and more angry and more ready. And we say her name on all the back blocks, and the neighbors cheer for her, because she is so obviously still alive.

4.

The old land sneaks up on me here and there. Every so often, I wail for Latasha Harlins, and for my brother cut down by vatos on Orange Avenue. Every so often, I find myself at the edge of the LA River blindly wailing, Bloody Mary.

Here the city I loved moves under me. The old lesbian bar, Sisters, fades into time, the place I learned old dykes survived, so too would I. And Elena's Soul bar smolders in the ashes of The Barn. And the free Greyhound to Atlantic City's been rerouted. The crisis nursery has been sold. And the jerk chicken man of Cedar Park been shut down. And all these memories saved my life.

5.

What I'm saying is I am running to where I am now. Across the wet grass of Malcolm X Park barefoot at dusk, away from the crisis response center and the squad car, Across the Old South Street Bridge, down endless wooded trails looking for clues left behind by teenagers living in the laundry room of our apartment building. They say in permanent marker graffiti'd to a basement wall: *It's warm down here*, and *You'll never find me*, and *Thank you!*

Sorrow for the Cobbs Creek Trees lost to a Golf course who watched over me in torturous nights as I mended the new wounds and the old ones, and made impossible decisions about living or dying. The tree line is a Black giant at night, steadfast breathing with me, and keeping me from the edges of their own cliffs, whispering wait wait wait, wait til the morning.

Now, the skeleton of my sibling, in piles of lumber, 100 acres of Kin cut clear and you can see 69th Street Station and the naked railway wires and lights and all its spindly machinations clear from Haverford Avenue.

I owe them a song at least, for all the dreams of future their leaves gave me. For the promise of sustenance, I dreamt of buried onions in the trails behind the apartment buildings and recounted these visions as me and the old dog found a way through the rocky banks of sparkling water. For prophecy of home, abundance, and kinship.

Today my child calls that dog an ancestor as we collect good rocks for skipping while the soft water laps at the pools of mud that collect gnats and mosquitos. And the hum of growth sings to us under the sway of limbs, and in the beat of wings.

[1]   *A kwe-kwe² is a Guyanese pre-wedding celebration.*

[2]   *The FAFSA³ is the Free Application for Federal Student Aid, a form that determines a student's eligibility for federal aid to attend college, university, or other secondary education institutions in the United States.*

[3]   *The M.O.V.E bombing[4] was an incident where then Philadelphia Mayor John Street ordered the firebombing of the Black radical organization M.O.V.E, killing most members of the family, including five children.*

#

Experiences of disposability: Discussion questions

Find the complete Surplus Person's Experience Survey in the Learning Opportunities section of this book, pg. [x].

1.   From your perspective as a care worker, mental health professional, and/or person in recovery, can you identify experiences where you felt dehumanized, disposable, or expendable? Reflect on one or more of these experiences. Include the institutional backdrop of these experiences, and any other details that contextualize your experience. Be sure to examine cultural institutions like "the nuclear family" as well as traditional systems if relevant.

2.   If you hold experiences of disposability, how do you manage those experiences today? Do you hide it from coworkers, from partners, from friends? Do you pretend to have resources that you don't have? How often do you do this?

3.   How would you describe the effects that being deemed disposable has had on your life? If you have not encountered disposability first hand, what have your interactions been like with disposable or "surplus people"? Describe your interactions and reactions to these encounters.

4. Can you imagine a future where you might be considered disposable? Or a future where currently disposable people are seen as valuable?

Examine your answers for points of intersection and solidarity with others who may encounter overwhelming feelings of helplessness, nihilism, and hopelessness. Examine your answers and experiences for areas of growth, change, and challenge to the status quo that identifies those of us as expendable.

2
DSM215 solutions

This chapter outlines the recent history of Deep Space Mind 215 and its projects, as well as emerging foundational frameworks informed by the grassroots work of Deep Space Mind 215 in local neighborhoods.

#

DSM215 background and manifesto

Background

Deep Space Mind 215 in its current iteration was born out of necessity in 2020 during the COVID-19, when a number of existing citywide issues related to collective health and quality of life hit a breaking point at the same time. While formal psychiatric, social service, education, and housing institutions struggled to meet the needs of local Philadelphians, the city saw an explosion of neighbor-driven initiatives to improve and protect each other outside of institutions.

Between 2020 and 2021, Rashni and Mel connected to establish practical, flexible mechanisms for community mental health support, including mutual aid for those facing houselessness, discord-based suicide prevention, and a youth public arts project around youth futurisms in mental health.

Deep Space Mind 215 has had many journeys since its first iterations as an Afrofuturist community art workshop in 2015. The workshop was designed to help participants celebrate their unique psychic experiences outside of Western conceptions of "mental health." Rashni was awarded a Blade of Grass Fellowship for Socially Engaged Art in 2019 to expand the series locally.

Today, Deep Space Mind 215 exists at the end of a successful, meaningful pilot project in its partnership with Pentridge Children's Garden and would like to mark this time period as a point of reflection and wisdom gathering after four years of direct community dialogue, planning, and action.

Deep Space Mind 215 statement of intent

We aim to celebrate Black madness, neurodiversity, and lived experience of mental health challenges and institutionalization as a powerful resource and source of wisdom, and a necessary ingredient for a community built with resilience and wellness in mind. This means coming together with our eyes set on peership and solidarity.

We share space with the intention of equity, the belief that everyone has a skill to share at their individual capacity, a history requiring us to hold a sense of sonder for both our collective and individual experiences and knowledge.

We see payment, compensation, and mutual benefit as a recognition of the labor our bodies take on when we use our own selves to promote the healing of other selves. We respect survivors for this skill and wisdom in the context of late capitalism.

We celebrate with libations and camaraderie, fanning the other ways of knowing and being, deemed as madness and pathology, that require dowsing out or placation by industries who capitalize off of our individual and collective sickness.

We prove that WE know what's best for ourselves.

We mourn those we lost also with libations and celebration, because a life is well lived if anytime spent attempting collective liberation. We become the human archive, with stories, having been witness to each other's lives.

Emerging DSM215 commitments

- Practicality, Critical Need, and Responsiveness

  Deep Space Mind 215 in its current iteration was born in out of necessity in 2020 during the COVID-19, in memory of that experience, and the legacy of Black health workers throughout history who created systems of care out of practical need. We want to continue mechanisms to stay in sync with local community need, acknowledging the city's chronic history of housing injustice, reliance on carceral institutions and systems, and slow moving ineffective bureaucracy that often works in antithesis to the safety and well-being of Black families and communities.

- Self-Determination Autonomy and Respect

  Compensation, mutual respect, no hierarchies with neighbors, leadership development among those with lived experience, building peer-led space, structure, and frameworks of understanding to drive narrative change in the mental health field of practice.

- Roots in Afrofuturist, Ancestral, and Sci-fi Practice

    Remembering our roots in ancestral, artistic, and Afrofuturist practice—unique perspective allows for local wisdom to prevail, and for dialogue in Black spaces that is relevant and reflexive to local interests and culture. Centering storytelling and futurist practice, including collective visioning and art-making. Centering intergenerational practice and the transmission of ancestral stories and strategies for survival. Commitment to creating a future-present where Black, queer, poor, mentally ill, and otherwise marginalized people can live with joy.

- Restorative Practice

    Ongoing education, movement building, training around restorative, ancestral ways of community practice, organization building, and community facilitation. Promoting repair, responsibility, relationships, and respect.

- Centering Lived Experience, Recovery, and Peership Models

    Centering and developing strategies for living and interdependence for those living with mental health challenges, centering disability justice tenets, i.e. community inclusion, participation, leadership. Include harm reduction for mental health challenges, substance use, and navigating systems of violence. Learning from Black Healing Experiences, and building a study around what allows these experiences to occur.

- Direct Community Dialogue

    Practitioners ARE community members; we are IN community, not working with a community. We aim to reduce barriers, making it regular practice to dialogue and build with neighbors in peership, and to be responsive to the needs of our community as we encounter overlapping synergies and values. We consider ongoing development of best practices for safer boundaries, and strong social-emotional skills in intergenerational, intersectional community engagement.

#

Defining the Black healing experience: Rashni Stanford
House of Umoja and the healing nature of circularity

In 2022, I had the sacred experience of visiting with Queen Mother Falaka Fattah in West Philadelphia at House of Umoja, a nonprofit that mentors Black youth and has weathered over 50 years of serving a city dealing with community violence and neglect. As I navigated transitioning out of working at a local drop-center for youth in foster care, as well as rapidly scaling up the work of Deep Space Mind 215 with Mel, I had taken on some freelance journalism work with the anti-carceral news publication *The Appeal.* While I felt my energy and hope flagging after two and a half years of tireless COVID-era work at an agency contracted by the city's Child Welfare system to protect and support our city's system-involved youth, learning about hyperlocal solutions with a real history in bringing results helped to refill my cup, and get the gears in my head turning about next steps for DSM215.

I listened to the origin story of House of Umoja, and of Queen Mother Fattah's early commitment to journalism and authentic Black storytelling around gun and youth violence at the time. Queen Mother Fattah and her late husband David Fattah along with House of Umoja are known to be responsible for brokering a ceasefire in 1974 between warring street gangs, called the

Imani Pact (Stanford, 2022). Today House of Umoja manages the Umoja Youth Peace Corps, an initiative that trains and employs local young people to support their community in maintaining peaceful relationships with one another, and making positive contributions to their community. The Umoja Peace Corps does this through conflict resolution and restorative practice train-ings, financial literacy, media, and technology training as well as opportunities to connect with Black tech and community lead-ers through field trips and events.

Before the non-profit, however, Queen Mother Falaka Fattah and her husband began their journey in community work when their son's friends let them know they didn't have a home to go to. In a radical act of community care, the Fattah's opened their home to these young men and allowed their stories to join their own.

Today at over 90 years old, Queen Mother Fattah continues to run communications for her organization, including Umoja Magazine, a "think tank of peace via accounts of lived experi-ences and collective wisdom" (Fattah, QMF, 2024). I was able to return to House of Umoja with my finished article and presented it to her and the rest of her staff, when they invited the piece to be published in an addition of Umoja Magazine. The circularity of this exchange felt immense and grounding for me.

The work of House of Umoja inspired me and was in direct dialogue with what DSM215's community had been working toward—a community-grown framework of neighborhood col-lectivity and mutual care. A method of problem-solving with roots in the practical traditions of our ancestors. After exploring other modalities of community intervention that centered lived experience, like peer support work or the local community health workers training, we decided to invest in restorative practices—a flexible, accessible model being undertaken throughout Philadelphia and the systems that involve so many of our neighbors based on mutual respect, trained trusted messengers, and collective dialogue and solution-building.

After holding an event at a local Black garden in North Philadelphia, we were introduced to the local Restorative Cities Initiative; to restorative practitioners at Eddie's House, a local youth homelessness organization; and Dynamic Justice Collective, an emerging restorative organization. From there we partnered with these groups to host the first paid restorative practice trainings for our community. Since then, we have hosted four restorative trainings, and trained 60 members of our community, paying them for their time.

We were even able to invite members of House of Umoja to that very first training and begin forming a connection outside of the walls of their organization.

This persistence of space and theme, the ability to return to each other and check-in on each other's progress in our shared visions of peace and self-sufficiency—these experiences have stayed with me as DSM215 continues to work to respond to community needs. Something about the circle speaks to me and my Blackness as a practitioner, especially one that has experienced the dehumanization of institutional "care."

House of Umoja is just one organization that we find ourselves revisiting and continuously building upon histories of connection and overlap. The ability to revisit each other is a privilege in

Black communities where erasure, displacement and gentrification are a norm. For someone like me who was raised in an urban area like Southern California that worked hard to scrub Black existence from its map, this persistence is infinitely calming and ultimately healing. For someone like me who was raised without consistent or present caregivers, connecting with a local elder with great capacity for intergenerational love and understanding has also brought me deep healing and rootedness.

So, my question has become, what other elements of group and community dynamics show themselves as effective and valuable in the fight against chronic trauma? What else can we begin to identify as invaluable to Black collective healing?

Defining a Black healing experience

One thing I know about the city of Philadelphia is that our neighbors don't like to waste their time. So drilling down for efficiency and practicality's sake on the types of collective experiences that feel valuable toward neighborhood health is important. It's also important that agencies and well-meaning clinicians find honest curiosity when their programming fails in Black communities, rather than quick pivots to the next trending intervention, defensiveness and community-blaming, or withdrawal of resources, care, or interest in a community because of an initial lack of engagement.

We at DSM215 have been curious about how to make the most of our time in community with our neighbors and have been asking the following questions throughout the course of our work: How can we gather community together in a way that feels valuable? How can we start to clearly define the value of gathering people with shared lived experience of mental health challenges, trauma, or neurodiversity to solve community wellness issues? What is it about trusting lived experience that is so valuable? How can we explore it with the gravity it deserves and release it from the prison of grant writing language and nonprofit box-checking? And ultimately: How do we know that we are experiencing a community dynamic or curating a community space that is good for us, healing us?

Afrofuturist neuropsychologist Dr. Tanisha Hill talks about the neurocircuitry of Black hope and begins to define the wild mindspace that produces what can seem like an impossible optimism and ingenuity within the Black community in the United States, driving us to resist the violence of institutional racism. After all it is a madness for our ancestors to have dreamt of freedom. In fact, drapetomania was once considered a psychiatric ailment, one of the first formal diagnoses in the United States, to crave freedom as a Black enslaved person. To that end, how can we hone in on elements of neighborhood spaces that promote the growth of collective trust, efficacy, and an increase in shared wellness.

I propose the framework of the Black Healing Experience as a container to begin to answer these questions. Black Healing Experiences are a nexus of ideas, attitudes, and experience that contribute to effective healing justice practices in Black communities. It is the phenomenology of wellness, trust, wholeness, healing, hope, and growth—a framework that would contribute on a neighborhood level to the great collective force that Dr. Hill-Jarrett calls "the Black Radical Imagination," which is comprised of (1) imagining alternative Black futures, (2) radical hope, and (3) collective courage (Hill-Jarrett, 2023). As Afrofuturists living with disabilities, we inject an anti-eugenicist, disability justice framework into this imagination, where Black madness is included and exalted in the legacies of Black radical futures and imaginations.

Beyond another behavioral inventory

Developing the construct of Black Healing Experiences has the unique opportunity to increase neighborhood-level access to collective efficacy, future orientation, connection, resource sharing, and space that can combat the collective effects of racialized, institutional trauma.

Rather than another clinical inventory or survey meant to label community members as damaged, or to assign short-lived futures to our neighborhoods, tools developed from the BHE framework would make sure to offer solutions and to set an experiential standard efficacy and self-assessment for neighborhood-level group work of any kind. It is a flexible concept that can be applied in clinical institutional settings to reestablish humanity with Black clients or in Black communities, or in care circles, family group decision-making, organizing spaces, or any other community-based gathering.

The groundbreaking ACEs study defined and surveyed Americans on their childhood experiences of trauma and uncovered the widespread nature of childhood trauma in this country. A high ACEs score has been shown to lead to poor health outcomes over the lifetime. Operationalizing the widespread, yet invisible problem of violence and trauma in the United States was undoubtedly valuable to the study of trauma under the medicalized model of mental health in the United States

However, a study of this construct and its limitations in actually proposing solutions to American collective trauma, or explaining how so many Americans, in spite of their trauma, managed to live full lives, eventually led to the development of the Positive Childhood Experiences survey. The PCE was seen as a much-needed expansion on ACEs, offering solutions to traumatic experiences, and a glimpse into personal resiliency and protective factors, rather than just scientific fate based on experiences that children cannot change. Children who experience high PCE scores, conversely, are buffered from the effects of trauma. While some of the PCE scale concerns factors within the child's home, many of the items concern access to community and cultural belonging and inclusion (Mitani et al, 2024).

Here is the opportunity to create similar definitions in defining positive elements of groups, communities, and neighborhood spaces that can encourage collective wellness in Black neighborhoods. Other communities in need of collective strength and efficacy can do similar work to elaborate on their own community's Healing Experiences and the elements that seem to be valuable in those locales and shared experiences.

Observed ingredients to support Black healing experiences from DSM215's early practice

Connection and vulnerability

+laughter, diversity of emotions and energies represented
+witnessing, acknowledgment, truth, reconciliation. accessibility to different minds and ages, perspectives, or strong advocacy for self at different ages.

+familiarity—straight talk reality checks with love, sharing secrets, holding, relating.

+mistakes, wounds, and risks are equally welcome and distributed synchronicities

+witnessing, hearing, silence, listening

+sharing of emotions without punishment, dispersal of emotion/energy shared among the group

+shared risk-taking, shared stakes

Practicality

+practicality, directness, and Black honesty—effectiveness/organicness

+authenticity

+self building and affirming

+resource sharing

+Time not wasted, economically and practically valuable

Local, living wisdom, history, and inter-generational dialogue

+the persistence preservation of connections, healing sites, histories

+circularity, relationships with people, sites, and communities are revisited with new growth and conduits of knowledge sharing

+rootedness, present and potential

+accountability "tell you about yourself" grounded, rooted a mirror

+intergenerational—restoring kinship, role of elders and historical context

+collective efficacy, ancestral, community strategies shared among neighbors

+staying power, non-extractive, and local

Futurity, spirituality, and creative power

+futurity, hope, radical imagination. collective creativity, energy for solution-making

+natural world, acknowledgments of connecting to land and body

+creative power, the collective imagination—storytelling, art-making, meaning-making

+divinity-sharing divine or transcendent experiences

Narrative change and justice

+rejection of dehumanizing lenses bravery and energy to do the work

+accessible and representative in the moment of that inclusivity

+A black disability justice rooted in culture

#

Opportunities in the Rubble: Discussion questions

Today, we observe global shifts in power, conceptions of truth, and beliefs in solidarity and basic humanity. Let us examine the rubble for solutions we can work toward in our current reality.

1. If you have ever worked for or received services from a social service, psychiatric, or healthcare institution [whether for self or a loved one], can you identify any moments of joy, authenticity, humanization, or effectiveness that have stuck with you? Describe these moments.

2. Who was present? What was the setting? What resistance to dehumanization did you or others enact?

3. How important is the neighborhood environment in building wellness for its residents?

4. What neighborhood structures have you found to promote wellness in your own life? It could be a treasured playground, rec center, or dance club. Describe the space, the people, and the elements that were most life-giving.

5. How have you observed disparities in neighborhood infrastructure? Can you identify how built space and neighborhood assets impact a community's ability to gather, problem solve, get to know each other, or celebrate together?

6. For those who are mental health professionals, do you see opportunities to support organic neighborhood wellness beyond your professional duties? Does it require bureaucratic resistance? What is the value of this resistance?

7. What is it about trusting lived experience that is so valuable?

8. How do we know healing is happening, or a space is open to healing connections?

3
Interviews

This chapter consists of dialogue with local neighbors who have worked alongside Deep Space Mind 215 in recent years, and the lived experience they bring to the work of their city, as well as the impacts DSM215's neighborhood-based modality has had on their work and their well-being.

#

Ms. Carol is a retired corporate logistics manager but a fiction writer at heart. Her family has been in the Cedar Park neighborhood for five generations at 50th Florence Ave. She lives in her grandmother's house. Each time Rashni and I visit, Carol greets us with libations, as she goes on about all the rent parties, and how her grandmother ran a speakeasy in the 1960s and 1970s. The house's weathered wood and crown molding tells stories of epic domino and card games with tobacco smoke in the air serving as a sign of good times.

#

Carol writes poems about love and forgiveness, archiving her daily moments riding the trolley to and from work, or the grocery, seeing past lovers and old friends. Her poetry and stories are a living archive to this historically Black west Philadelphia neighborhood. Carol's recounting of history pays homage to her legacy and to the many hands that have come before her to tend this community of neighbors, for better or worse.

#

In our time together Carol admits to not having the greenest of thumbs, yet that she's a "forever learner still grasping what the earth is." She tells us about her memories of the matriarchs of the family, how her grandmother and mother preserved things, tended plants in the house, and all around the backyard. Carol's kin came up from Clint, South Carolina before she was born, bringing with them many traditions of the south. "Food as medicine," Carol reflects on her own health, later in life appreciates being taught some of the old ways. She admits that she now understands the importance of passing these ways down to the grandchildren and the work of preserving the stories of the people who were once here.

Nana, Carol's grandmother, had roses and azalea bushes on the front porch. Her near-corner tri-story West Philadelphia house was considered as a "curb appeal house." A shed kitchen was tightly tucked in the back alley, where she grew peppers, okra, onions, collards, tomatoes, basils, and something called a rutabaga. Growing along the perimeter of the house was a fox grapevine, cascading in the back of the house. Nana preserved grape jelly and made sticky fermented grape wine. A friend to the grapevine was a mulberry bush. Nana used its berries to dye things and the leaves, to beat the dirt out of Mr. Freddie's, her grandfather, work shirts. Carol remembers being mystified by the whole process. Mr. Freddie would come and cut the trees in the winter, and Nana would begin making her preserves. Nana had many different jobs, but one thing she was passionate about was feeding her family and working as a chef at Linton's Restaurant at Broad and Wallace. Carol tells us about how during the winter holidays she'd help her Nana haul sweet potatoes across town from Mr. Linton's to bake the restaurant's famous sweet potato pies. Her mother was the harvester of the family. Carol reflects and now understands the symbiotic relationships it takes to grow food. "Everybody has a role to play."

\#

Today Carol still grows beautiful bright blush pink and red peonies in her front yard. Her career led her to Germany for many years till she returned to her home at 50th and Florence, and eventually taking over the Pentridge Children's Garden in 1992. Her daughter started her own family, and Carol was to be the new matriarch of the generation. PCG was a gathering space for families to come, convene, and grow things together. Carol recalls so many memories of her grandchildren being young learners and garden helpers throughout the years, as many families came and went. Some families were displaced during the crack epidemic in the late eighties and early nineties. Carol remembers coming home from abroad to a place that was less familiar. Disintegration of the West Philly community had taken its grip on its people. Houses sat for decades to follow, left to the process of dilapidation. As resources slowly receded in the community along with tremendous loss of loved ones, families struggled to keep their homes, many choosing to sell or leave, marking the familiar process of gentry[5] or tactical urbanism[6].

\#

She remembers the M.O.V.E bombing with tears in her eyes, and how time stopped as the ground lifted and shook. This was just another telling moment where she learned a lesson about how all your "skin folk ain't your kinfolk," as the first Black mayor of Philadelphia gave the order for the bomb to be dropped on the back of 62nd and Osage Ave less than a mile radius from her Cedar Park home. "That voice has stayed with her throughout the years," Carol states. For her that day is a reminder that connecting with her affinity community and deep efforts toward understanding one another's differences, not as means of tolerance, but as what keeps us alive, thriving as a community.

#

Pentridge Children's garden embodied - Mel Brown

I stand at the iron gate. It's funny because I can never remember the code, so I have to carry my phone with me and find the last message where I would've shared (fades out) the code to someone.

I scan the grass, looking at the beds, the dirt, thinking about the archival footage of the garden, from forever ago, or what feels like it. I scan my memory of that footage, comparing it to where my feet are placed, in real life, trying to re-create or adjust the two images on top of each other. Blanche Epps' voice approaches me, with her criteria for what makes a good gardener. She tells me stories of her family migrating to Philadelphia from the south after the First World War, bringing gardening with them, while expressing the dire need for growing food, and how in her time they lacked access to fresh vegetables in the city (Philly Folklore Project, 2015).

This is still a place of rest, even after its grounds shook that spring day, May 13, 1985. Even further I can imagine coming here after a long day of work, finally resting my body underneath the apple tree, grazing on fox grapes. In this garden, man created shade for relief from the oppressive sun, to escape from being witnessed, seen, or questioned while at rest, as if caught resting, while Black was proof of being lazy, second class, or lesser than. I think of the brilliance of Tricia, The Nap Ministry, how today we rest from some of the same battles fought back then, but in new ways, and how the dirt carries so much of the history in it (Hersey, 2022). How it gives back to us, and how the ground beneath us carries our bodies from one place to the next. Wondering if it could ever belong to anyone, or if we belong to it. How would that change things?

Today, there remains that apple tree, a fig tree, a pomegranate tree, and somewhere hidden an olive tree. The rose of Sharon greets you at the front of the garden, spilling over the gate, blooming its pink blossoms faithfully each year. The tale is that the fig tree that announces itself long before entering the garden is the largest living fig tree in the city's numerous arboretums, farms, (fades) orchards, gardens....

#

Avani interview - Rashni Stanford

Avani Alvarez is the current executive director of Creative Resilience Youth [CRY], a youth-led initiative committed to justice in youth mental health care, as well as a member of Stewardship Council at Pentridge Children's Garden, the pilot site of DSM215's emerging restorative neighborhood mental health practice. Avani is rooted along with their mother in West Philadelphia and, along with being a youth advocate, is a multidisciplinary artist, whose work seeks to stimulate introspection in the viewer.

Avani first encountered Deep Space Mind 215 in 2020 as a senior in high school when they participated in the Young Futurist Study Series, a virtual synergy facilitated by DSM215 between the youth-led art-making initiatives Young Artist Program and Creative Resilience Youth. The Young Futurist series grew out of a mutual interest between the three groups to creatively and directly address the critical mental health needs of Philly youth during the onset of the COVID pandemic. It consisted of Zoom study sessions where I led youth and adult allies of both collectives through Afrofuturist perspectives in youth mental health, youth organizing, and art-based movement practice.

The series culminated in the summer of 2021 when the youth participants produced a collaborative public art exhibition called Roots Before Branches *at the Cherry Street Pier* (Rauch, 2021; Given, 2021). *The exhibition offered the public glimpses of youth futurisms that imagined worlds of safety, memorial, and justice for those with disabilities, the environment, and young people, as well as protection from racial, political, and sexual violence.*

The exhibition also marked the first collaboration between myself and Mel, who as co-founder of the Young Artist Program was in the midst of running programming with their young people during the onset of COVID-19. It was during this collaboration that Mel and I began building DSM215 to what it is today.

It has been a joy to reconnect with Avani four years after our first meeting to catch up with them about their journey as a young community practitioner and the ways their practice has been impacted by Deep Space Mind 215's ethos.

Rashni *When did you first encounter DSM215 and what was that like? Where were you in your career and interests at that time?*

Avani   The first time I came in contact with DSM was I think through Andrea Nan, who invited myself and a few other youth to a training, we were all on Zoom, taking this training you guys were doing. It was definitely during COVID in 2020.

R   *Was it the Young Futurist Study Series?*

A   Yes! The Young Futurist Study Series. I was working and I was a student. I was an essential worker at the time. It was certainly a needed time to have that series in my life for sure. I was an essential worker at Sprouts and I went to high school at CAPA. And before the pandemic really hit, I would just saunter over to my job right next door and change into my uniform and get to work.

R   *How did you get in contact with CRY [Creative Resilience Youth]?*

A   I got into contact with CRY through Michele Delgado when I was in Teen Photo at the Philadelphia Photo Arts Center. Michele had emailed myself and a few other youth to apply to this thing. It's funny, it was supposed to be an 8-week program, and 7 years later here we are still.

R   *How does it feel to still be connected with CRY today?*

A   It's a really amazing feeling. I don't think I would have made it very far in life and living if I hadn't found this program. MY family has always been really immersed in mental health struggles. No one really addressed it or knew how to address it. In seeing all that as a teenager, I just didn't want to claim anything, I didn't want to claim being an artist, or any sort of leadership. They helped me tackle my understanding around my family dynamics and my family's relationship with mental health, as well as my own relationship with mental health, as well as my own relationship with being an artist, a teaching artist, and organizer.

R   *Where were you living at the time?*

A   I was living in West Philly. The house that I'm Zooming you from now is where we were living, I'm house sitting for my mom in Cobbs Creek.

R   *What were your interests when you got in contact with DSM215?*

A   I was really interested in being some sort of art director. I wanted to own a gallery, I wanted people to share their art there, or be a creative director of some kind because I was really good at helping people as opposed to my own creative projects. I wanted to be a huge support to other people and the arts. I was playing with the idea of becoming a therapist because of what I had seen in my family. I would love to be someone for other people to talk to because I saw that's what was needed in my own family. But as a teen, I wanted to do more art.

R   *How did your involvement with CRY evolve into more than an
     8-week program?*

It was a little bit of both. [I was naturally engaging with CRY]
and with the Young Futurist Study Series, I realized this is so
much bigger than I originally thought it was and I want to
keep being a part of this world of advocacy and organizing,
and it's interesting, it tickles my fancy. All of the people we
were introduced to through CRY, we were like "We don't want
this to stop, we want to keep learning about all these things
and teaching our peers about."

R   *I remember your art piece for the Roots Before Branches
     exhibition, and how much interaction your art piece had gotten
     at the Cherry Street Pier. Can you tell us more about it?*

A   I still have all the responses I got from that. I keep them in
     a safe box. That was an amazing project. I had asked a lot
     of questions around introspection and loneliness because it
     was the pandemic. I knew my experience during the pan-
     demic. I was incredibly lonely and I experienced multiple
     transformations, some for better some for worse. The project
     was a manifestation of my curiousness. I wanted to ask "How
     are you guys doing in the midst of all this?" It was really beau-
     tiful the responses I got. Some people answered the prompt
     and were very "Here's question 1, here's question 2" but some
     people answered in such a way like this profound expression
     of, "I am lonely and I am longing for community." I remember
     when I moved to New York, because at the time, we set up
     the exhibition, I moved and I had to travel back from New York
     to be a part of the show. And I remember having to   collect
     everything reading them back in my tiny, tiny bedroom in
     New York and just sobbing from all the beautiful messages.

Because NYC, because I had just moved to NYC at that time. I felt so connected to these people I didn't know the names and faces of. The way that it was set up was the one side of the wall had all these questions, and the other side there was paper to write on, and everyone had the chance to see what people wrote and to post their own pieces.

R   *What was that experience like to interact back then, to be with CRY but in collaboration with another youth-led program, YAP, and with DSM215? It was during COVID, we were all under lockdown and had a figure out a way to get this thing off the ground.*

A   It was really interesting. I remember I knew some of the folks in CRY, and I know we couldn't be as in tune with one another because of the pandemic. It was the first time CRY did a collaborative exhibition too, it was a new thing for all of us in a lot of ways. I remember how much joy I felt seeing everyone's art pieces. These people i been connecting with over Zoom, some people I never seen their faces before. And seeing the art they created was just so … I don't even know if there were words to describe how I felt walking around Cherry Street Pier, seeing everything that everyone made. especially from YAP[1]. it was really inspiring for me especially as a young person at that time because i felt very lonely, very existential, I'll be in NYC going to college, it's not really real cause it's COVID. Newly coming into my identity as an artist and the type of art I wanted to make. And seeing how other people made their art and express themselves was inspiring and reaffirming.

R   *What happened with school in New York?*

A   I ended up dropping out of school because I'm poor, and it wasn't what I expected it to be. I was going to Parsons at the time, I was really excited to go, it was the only school I applied to, […] and I got in. But the learning experience was not worth the tuition. Despite having to pay for school myself, they didn't really give much assistance. I was like "I can't afford to be here and it's not worth it, so I'm out." Then I was just in New York working. I came back to Philly in April of 2022. I was only out in New York for a year.

R   *What was it like re-entering the city?*

A   It was so comforting because the support systems I knew were all here, not in New York. I was out on my own having fun with new friends, working and struggling. My time in New York was a lot of struggle. And coming back to Philly it was like "Oh my gosh I don't have to struggle anymore, and I'm surrounded by people who love me so much." I moved in with my closest friends at the time straight from a bad living situation in New York. It was the perfect landing to come back to. Then I got more heavily involved with CRY once I came back to Philly.

R   *Were you able to make a living reconnecting with CRY?*

A   CRY is completely sustaining my life right now, and i am eternally grateful because in this work it can be really hard to live off of doing this. I'm very fortunate that we have been able to pay everyone that we've come in contact with. It's important to pay people for their time

R   *How would you describe your practice today?*

A   My practice now is interesting. In the community I really like intergenerational healing and community building. I love connecting people with other people, I love to provide access. I am in a very privileged position in this space to be able to provide access to those resources. I'm like "What resources do we have, who wants it and how do we get it to them in a way that makes sense?"

R   *Fast forward to now, I know this summer you completed our Restorative Neighborhood Mental Health Training at Pentridge Children's Garden. What was that training like for you?*

A   That training was a part of really huge shift in my life this year, which thank you guys so much. There was so much beautiful energy in the room and so many amazing people in the room that i met, that have expanded my perspective of what it means to be in community with people, the different the realities that can be. Not the possibilities, but the actual realities. Seeing people actually living it or working to live in that was powerful and inspiring.

One practice you emphasized a lot which I held near and dear to my heart was circling, how circling was a huge part of community, and a huge part of coming together and problem-solving. You talked about problem-solving as a community especially around mental health crisis instead of calling the police. There are so many people who are like "ACAB[2], abolish the police," but there's never a next step of like what do we do as an alternative to that and I don't think that's talked about enough.

There was a whole session where we were dreaming up what fruitful and safe communities would look like us as mad, BIPOC, queer, trans, neurodivergent people. It was both so beautiful to see this and be like, "Gosh this would be so perfect if we were able to make this happen," but also very disheartening knowing all the systems that make it so that can't be the case. Then inspiring again to see what we can do in our own communities to get us closer to those realities. Got me thinking a lot about public health and urban design justice. I thought a little bit about design justice because mentors and friends have been involved in that. I never really put it as part of my ethos I guess, but after the training, I realize I can be a part of that movement and help drive it.

R   *How have these trainings affected you or your practice? Have any of the Afrofuturist elements felt relevant to you?*

A   The first encounter I ever had with y'all in the Young Futurist Study Series, was my introduction me to afro-futurism. I grew up with a grandmother who was very pro-Black and who did things with the Black Panther Party, but she never talked to me about afro-futurism, but you were the first people to introduce me to that. Experiencing that in both trainings has been so amazing. It's helped me understand how to decolonize a lot of ways, especially coming into a position of leadership. I want to stay true to these morals and beliefs, and a lot of that flows through with afro-futurism and advocating for my folks. So, leading with that. I'm thinking about how at PCG we're not calling it an advisory board, and we're taking a different approach by calling it the "stewardship council," all of these ways we are breaking down all the roots of this stuff. It effects how I show up as an educator, human being with my friends and a family.

R   *How does your community practice show up in your family dynamic?*

A   Oh man, it's funny you ask. My grandmother is still in California. We moved here in 2013. Since I was a kid, I've been a mediator between my grandmother and my mom and other people, and as I've gotten older, did stuff with CRY, DSM215, I've learned to understand my grandma better. She's not just a crazy lady who's religious. She's a very traumatized and mentally ill person who needed different supports and different level of care and consistency in order to open up. me and my mother's dynamic has changed in a huge way in some good ways and some bad ways. by learning all these tools and knowledge and applying that to my own mental health and relating to my grandmother, educating my mother on mental health in general because she wasn't the most understanding in general. that helped her understand her mother better, so it's tightened up our immediate family unit.

R   *It sounds like Intergenerational issues that came before you have affected you.*

A   Yeah, my mom and grandmother always say Avani is the oldest, my mom's the youngest, and grandma is second youngest. They call me the intergenerational family curse breaker. It's sweet but also heavy to hold.

R   *Is that a role you would have willingly chosen if you had the choice?*

A   I would have still chosen that role. My mom has done a great job of saying you're young you don't have to hold all of this, but I am saying it's ok. It's a lot but I'm not holding it alone. i would have still chosen to impact my family in this way. Do I wish there were some minor tweaks? Absolutely. But I can't see a world where I wasn't in this position with my family.

R   *What support would you have liked to see for yourself in your life as a young Black person, and community practitioner?*

A   I would love to have seen more understanding and a willingness, especially in community organizing and building.

Everyone is afraid to be wrong and make mistakes. And being gentle and compassionate. Less shame. The hardest part of my mental health journey is that I saw shame at the root of a lot of it within myself that was learned from my family members. They didn't know how to deal with their mental health other than shame. Shame within themselves, upon other people going through similar things. That got very internalized and I wish there was a lot less. Destigmatizing it completely, and coming from a place of curiosity instead "That's different and weird, ew."

R   *How would you describe some of the lived experiences you and your family held in clinical, or "Western" terms?*

A   With my grandmother I was worried that she was bipolar or a paranoid schizophrenic. Now that's changed, my whole family struggles with a spectrum of Obsessive Compulsive Disorder [OCD]. A lot of the women and femmes in my family specifically. Either OCD in terms of hoarding, or in terms of everything needs to be a particular way.

R   *Do you have any alternative or ancestral explanations for your experiences?*

A   My mom is very logical whereas my grandmother is very illogical when it comes to being severely mentally ill. And my mom was a huge catalyst for change. It couldn't have gone any other way—if she hadn't been the way she was, I wouldn't have been the way I was. I wouldn't have been a curse breaker if it hadn't been for what my mom had been working toward. The way that we went about breaking the curse was different, where I saw things far beyond my immediate family unit, whereas my mom only saw it in my grandmother. Because that's really all we had, we were very disconnected from my family on this side. Now that we're all here, I'm recognizing patterns, and she's recognizing it too, so a lot of perspectives are changing. I don't know what you would call that.

R   *How things showed up are how they needed to show up, rather than getting rid of something problematic.*

A   My family for so long operated on "getting rid of what's problematic." That's a huge reason my grandma is the way that she is. It was just like get rid of, push to the side, ignore, move forward. my grandma didn't have the tools to go against that grain, but also knew it didn't feel right, so she would just run away. She has been all around the country not just because she liked sight-seeing. She was run away from traumatic event after traumatic event after traumatic event, and not knowing how to communicate that or what to do about that, other than to just get away from it.

I think hopefully, between the three of us, that was the end of that. My mom came around and that was a challenge to that, and when I came around that was another challenge to that.

R   *Now it seems you have some rootedness in Philadelphia. Do you have the same tendency to run as your grandmother?*

A   My mom and I both have talked about how we both need to be rooted and settled somewhere, which is funny thinking about how the woman who raised us is. I'm mostly just wanting to stay put somewhere and just make the best out of it. When we first moved here, we were originally in South Philly. And then my mom became a homeowner and bought this house here in Cobbs Creek. This is where we were, which is also so wild that she became a homeowner, it was incredible.

My mom spent so much time renting and my grandma never owned property so it was this thing. I never thought owning land was something for me to do. My mom always dreamt and had dreams she would own a home.

R   *Where were you born?*

A   I was born in California, and came here at 11 years-old. I hated the move, when I first came to Philly, I was like what is this tiny, dirty city, why are the houses so close together? where are the mountains, where is the nature? Why is everything concrete? I was so not used to it. I grew up in an apartment complex but also a few blocks from the mountains. It was a small town near the mountains, I had coyotes coming into the complex and I thought they were dogs. I was really used to being heavily immersed in nature, watching the stars, and the wildfires on the mountains. Moving to Philly was a really wild shock. We moved at night, so I couldn't see anything, and then the next morning, I was like, "What is this one-way street you speak of? Why are the houses so close together, why are the cars on the sidewalk?" We moved right to 30th and Tasker, before they put that dog park and started gentrifying.

R   *What have been challenges in your practice as someone with lived experience?*

A   On a personal level, especially with my history with my family, it's been really hard accepting help. I found it a serious challenge to advocate for myself and to accept help and community from other people. Learning how to be in community with other people was a real big stepping stone in my life, because I had been told my whole life that you need to figure that out on your own, both from my family members, and from the world. Confronting that head on, I was like that doesn't feel right to me, caring for your community is caring for yourself. But it took a lot of learning. I am still learning how not to be a sour lone wolf about needing help or being reminded to rest. Remembering my humanity was a huge challenge. Remembering my humanity as a young, queer neurodivergent, person of color, because from so young I was worked to the bone at Sprouts, and in retail. There was a point in high school where I was like this is gonna be the rest of my life, working doing hard labor in grocery stores and destroying my body, waking up at the ass crack of dawn, going home and seeing no one.

And now we're here, so yipee!

R   *What can you see for your future right now?*

That's a hard question, because the future could be so many things. The immediate future for me, my grandmother is going to be moving back to Philadelphia. It is something that we've been working toward for 12 years, before we even left. It's the end of a huge cycle in my family. I think it's going to be a big period of change for all of us.

Further down the line, I see myself taking on a caretaker role but not for an individual. I have to remind myself not to lose myself in that. I see that being a challenge for me. I'm not losing myself in that role that I assigned myself to.

My grandmother is from Philadelphia. Our family started in Philly up Ogontz [3]. She left when she was young, but has only been back once to visit us after we first moved here and hasn't been back since.

R   *What will your care network look like with her here?*

A   I really don't know. I know it's going to be hard because Philly is a hard place for [my grandmother] to be in. It's hard to give in to the fact you are aging and need to be cared for in itself, let alone other issues my family has with asking for help in general. I think it's also going to bring my family closer together. We'll be like "Wait a minute she's coming back home we need to be prepared and celebrate her." It's a new glue which is exciting.

R   *What's one thing from this summer's training that stays with you?*

A   I remember one guy who had recently come to terms with his autism diagnosis, and it was around the same time I also realized "Oh shit I'm autistic!" And I remember how I was kinda eavesdropping on the conversation, because they were talking to you. I remember feeling so affirmed in that because I was like "Wow, we're all discovering this in their own pace." I was feeling some type of way, my friends would make jokes like "How did you not know blahblah. hearing someone else working through the same thing that I was, and we're both relating on the tests. We didn't realize neurotypical people didn't do this! There were a few pockets. I think a lot about the centerpiece we created. The image of that in the middle of the room always sticks in my mind.

R   *How do you know you're having a healing experience in this city?*

A   I know I've had a healing experience when I come back to my healing station and I'm not dissociating. When I have a healing experience, I come back feeling recharged, whereas with every other interaction I feel drained, a piece of social battery is taken out. In those moments when I come across people or events or a combination, and I don't feel that way,

I know something in me has shifted and clicked. I've experienced a lot with DSM215 in 2020 and 2021, and also through Pentridge Children's Garden, I experienced that too, me and my mom. It's a second recharge station, I go to the garden and wow it feels so good to be out here with these people, I could be here all night.

DSM is really good at, for example, when I come to an event and I'm in a dissociative state, something about what we do there pulls me out of it, which is really, really nice. I don't know what that is, I can't pinpoint it, but something in that it's very easy to pull me out of it to experience. I don't always come ready to experience.

#

Interview with Queen of Dynamic Justice Collective and Restorative cities initiative - Rashni Stanford

We were introduced to Queen-Cheyenne Wade (Queen) in 2022 when DSM215 embarked on a journey of learning and skill-sharing around Restorative Practices, following interest from our community. Queen, along with Marion Campbell of Eddie's House, and Reverend Donna Jones of the Restorative Cities Initiative, introduced our collective to the local restorative justice landscape. In Philadelphia, restorative practices, like circles and family group conferencing, have been integrated into juvenile and adult criminal legal systems, the child welfare system, and public schools to different degrees, with local practitioners often being tapped to fulfill those duties.

Queen is the co-founder of Dynamic Justice Collective and is a restorative and transformative justice practitioner. For the past seven years, she has worked with system-involved young people, families, and individuals using restorative practices through organizations such as Philadelphia's Restorative Cities Initiative, Youth Art & Self-Empowerment Project, HEART Cambridge, and more. Queen partnered with DSM215 at the outset of our restorative practice study, trained DSM215 staff, and supported us in training 30 other Philadelphians in restorative practice.

The onset of the pandemic exposed the deep fissures in the nation's child welfare and juvenile detention systems. Locally youth experiencing homelessness and foster care, as well as child deaths in foster care rose during that time, including the 2023 death of two-year-old Su'Layah Williams, which rocked our city. This interview takes place a month after this tragedy. Queen reflects on how restorative practice can support the safety of Black families outside the child welfare system.

\#

Rashni   *You recently trained staff of DSM215 in restorative practices and restorative circling, alongside your business partner, Ken Peeples. You described using restorative practices both within the existing child welfare system, as well as an alternative to that system. What has your direct experience been in utilizing restorative practice as a mechanism to support families?*

Queen   My mom lives with a chronic disability, and she created what our neighborhood needed in Cambridge, whether it was support groups for young moms, family dinners, or childcare collectives.

Seeing that growing up draws me to this work more, because what she did doesn't require mandated reporting, or a master's degree; to this day people tell me how it impacted them to be supported in circles outside the carceral system. I saw these things from a young age. I got to see kids and parents find solutions together.

R   *What do you see as the issue with how the current child welfare system operates?*

Q   The system doesn't care about child autonomy, or disabled parent autonomy, in my case or low-income autonomy. It actively works against how Black families naturally make decisions, how we engage in justice, which is in community with one another.

Mandated reporting theoretically is fine, but practically it's weaponized against Black, undocumented, and disabled families. As a youth, I've been stopped by therapists who were mandated reporters, so when I wanted to dig into family issues I couldn't. I didn't wanna get my family in trouble. Mandated reporting offers no solutions, and is a threat rather than something that will support youth and families with accountability and autonomy.

R   *What are the ways restorative practices can be used in this context to support Black families?*

Q   I have been part of a kind of restorative circle called Family Group 'Conferencing' that helps transform and restore family autonomy by coming together to make plans that work for them. It's a collective process that says, "Let's get people what they need in their words."

I've seen when community comes around a family, like in restorative circles, it helps avoid the need for reporting. So many entities want to tear kids away from being rooted in Black and indigenous communities. Also, because these systems view Black and Indigenous communities as something "unsafe" or "uncivilized." But in actuality, many communities have been kept alive only because of the systems we've created outside of the state systems forced upon us.

I don't want to apologize for abuse in our communities either, but even as a survivor of domestic violence, I didn't want to punish the person with pain from the carceral system. I wanted him to understand and take account for the pain he caused and take actions to make things right with me, my family and our community. Restorative conferencing always leads to more solutions because it is collaborative and invites all of those impacted to come together. I am thankful I had restorative circles and could access that with my parents. It was so much better than any court-ordered individual or group therapy.

Right now, in our current state, when there is a safety issue reported, there is one process for all cases, and limited options for a lot of different needs.

Circling and conferencing are also more flexible, and fit more kinds of needs, because it does not try to fit multiple conflicts into one solution. It fits in with family's lives and works to keep kids connected to communities, instead of snapping them out of it. Restorative justice offers proactive approaches to address harm as well. So that we are not only practicing these values of safety or autonomy when something is wrong, but all throughout our communities and homes. There are also community trainings, one-on-one, and mediation as other ways for communities to problem solve and connect.

R   *What do you hope for the future of restorative practices as a way to strengthen Black families and communities?*

Q   There's the opportunity to work with the whole community to bring a different version of accountability than the courts can accomplish on their own. I think everyone should experience or build skills with restorative practice. We need restorative child care collectives, parent support spaces, abolitionist spaces for youth. We need more places where we can experiment together with different forms of decision making, conflict resolution, and different shifts in power between youth and parents. We need to integrate history and memory into educating our community about restorative justice, and histories of colonization, and continue to make connections to our everyday experience.

[1]   Young Artist Program, a local youth-led arts group for LGBTQ young people

[2]   Popular saying "All Cops Are Bastards"

[3]   Ogontz[8] is a neighborhood in North Philadelphia

#

Community trust and connection readiness self assessment: Discussion questions

Developing trust within our city with neighbors and colleagues has been the result of long-term commitment to neighbors, willingness to persist through conflict and uncertainty, and a tendency to circle back in order to strengthen bonds and build on past collaborations and conversations. Social service and psychiatric industries often discourage organic community building in a professional context. Use these questions to examine ways trust and community building have been affected by the current state of social service and mental health care.

1. What institutions, bureaucracy, or other external barriers have stood in the way of working effectively and feeling authentically connected to community? To neighbors? To clients?

2. What elements of your experience have stood in the way of working effectively and feeling authentically connected to community? To neighbors? To clients?

3. What relationships to institutions, systems, or other spaces of power do I maintain that prevent me from connecting authentically to community?

4. What experiences do I have where I felt heard, witnessed, or truly collaborative? Were they in professional settings? Healthcare settings? Neighborhood settings? What elements of those experiences feel most valuable to me?

5.   What are ethics you hold around trust, commitment, and intimacy with your "community"? What have you learned from elders, peers, and ancestors about these bonds? How have modern media, digital communication, and political division affected these beliefs?

4
DSM215 syllabus and archive

The following materials are a collection of exercises, inspiration, and challenges to the mainstream medical model of mental health and treatment developed in dialogue with our community, and our own practice. Archival material collected here serves as a testament to the wisdom around mental health and wellness that exists in Black communities, and the ways non-traditional neighborhood spaces serve as conduits to healing and growth.

#

The sustainability project (urgent strategies for communities) - Mel Brown

During the COVID-19 Pandemic Mel Brown lived in the North Philadelphia area of the city of Philadelphia which was affected by the uprisings concurrently happening across the city. In that time, the housing crisis in Philadelphia continued to balloon which led to self determining camps to be erected in two parts of the city. These camps were able to temporarily suffice as a third space for radical action. In that time mutual

aid became common household language, Mel created a
syllabus for those called to self organize on the ground actions.

Training activities and resources (this can be printed and discussed as a group)

Acknowledgment of privilege:

- Why is intersectionality vital?
- What is solidarity?
- In what ways do we have cross solidarity?
- Unpacking the P (privilege) word-naming your privilege (not really, make a list)
  o What is earned privilege?
  o What is unearned privilege?
- What does it mean to be deserving of something?
  o What does that cost other people?
  o Why is the importance of transparency?
- What is autonomy?
  o What does it cost you?
  o Comparatively?
- What are you willing to lose, for the sake of others' liberation?

Addressing the individual and the community (answer and research these questions as a group)

- Can we acknowledge our humanity and extend this respect to others?

- o How do we be stewards to our own trauma while stewarding others?
- o It's not our fault, and it's our responsibility.
- How do we understanding conflict?
  - o Conflict model
  - o Resolution model
  - o Stages of change
- Blackfoot model of wellness and self actualization— Naamitapiikoan Blackfoot Influences on Abraham Maslow

How do we assess our individual needs and our needs as a community?

How do we enact self sustainability?

- COVID-19 taught us about labor?
  - o Locally
  - o Globally

How do we build sustainable communities amidst human warfare?

Actionable STEPS as a community:

Is there a call to action/cease fire?

- List of demands
- Funding for redevelopment
- Healing inner-communally
- Creation of Community Agreements
  - o Micro
  - o Meso
  - o Macro

- Creation of Community Accountability
  - o Micro
  - o Meso
  - o Macro

List of reading resources and DATA:

- **Police Abolition—A World Without Police-**http://aworldwithoutpolice.org/
- **White Supremacy a Study Guide-** http://www.cwsworkshop.org/PARC_site_B/dr-culture.html
- **Chicago Police Abolitionist Movement-** https://m.chicagoreader.com/chicago/police-abolitionist-movement-alternatives-cops-chicago/Content?oid=23289710
- **Alternative To the Police-** https://www.mcgilldaily.com/PoliceIssue/Restorative-Justice.html

History of American Abolition-

- **American Abolition 1787 to 1861-** https://drive.google.com/file/d/1-4aVnRafj12yu--YeDstJgto2EnXBLZF/view?usp=sharing

Self governing/determination communities-

- **White supremacy as a social construct-** http://www.cwsworkshop.org/PARC_site_B/dr-culture.html
- **Bhutan's Happiness measurement model "Beyond Measurement" Episode-** https://whyy.org/episodes/beyond-measure/

Mutual Aid Resources

- **Grocery Run Templet-** https://docs.google.com/spreadsheets/d/1D04DQFHdYTNvsOaBXj_-DsLL0SYIIzQZuw-u3JI_pFA/edit?usp=sharing
- **COVID19 Syllabus-** https://docs.google.com/document/u/0/d/1-IRVbz1nsBQJHcaCVh8QLRBiwj3cFT_bXSwmTNs_Hf0/mobilebasic

- **COVID-19 Racial Capitalism Study-** https://drive.google. com/file/d/1NyVbhNpNzVABUMOvfuodz89-sZ23opDo/ view?usp=sharing
- **Alternatives to DSM5/ Diagnostic to Disorders: The Power Threat Meaning Framework-** https://www.bps. org.uk/power-threat-meaning-framework
- **Mental Health Initiatives(management): DSM215 Co- op-**https://www.deepspacemind215.com/
- **Canned Responses For Black Folks-(mental health protection)-** https://hashtagprotectyourenergy.weebly. com/

Environmental Racism:
- **Flint Michigan-** https://drive.google.com/file/d/1zrlgcKfLq WeeoEBGQWExEYRifsneHBIk/view?usp=sharing

Critical Race Theory:
- **Critical Race Theory As a Tranformative Model of Teaching Diversity-** https://drive.google.com/file/d/1j9ai_ QpzOASO--etAaQf7Cpte2jrsdkY/view?usp=sharing
- **Anti Asian Violence and Black—Asian Solidarity Today-** https://youtu.be/MGpo9419ViE

Findings from DSM215's first restorative neighborhood mental health training and other activities - Rashni Stanford

#

Collective notes from DSM215's first restorative neighborhood mental health training, summer 2024

With gratitude for the Philadelphians who engaged with us with their whole hearts for three powerful days, and offered their experiences, strategy and future vision.

These notes are compiled from feedback of the participants of DSM215's three day Restorative Neighborhood Mental Health training offered for the first during our 2024 Land and Wellness Summer Series.

Participants are neighbors with lived experience of mental health challenges who seek training in restorative practice and strategies for addressing mental health, and who are ready to practice these skills in their communities. Participants represented the city's youth organizers, people in recovery, people re-entering community after incarceration, environmental, food, and land justice practitioners, researchers, social workers, artists, queer and trans communities, and parents.

While DSM215 has partnered with local practitioners to offer community trainings on restorative practice before, this session marks the launch of our original restorative practice training with a particular emphasis on collective mental health care, community care planning, the role of dysregulation in movement work, and more.

Community Agreements:
- Honoring your body especially your nervous system
- Respect each other's space and orientations and character
- Listen to understand
- Respect boundaries
- Moments for pause
- Make use of COVID resources
- Show up courageously—challenge is ok and answers are not always clear
- Open-mindedness—attempt to understand
- Assume positive intentions
- Respect mental space of others, and don't take it personal
- Celebrating madness
- Misunderstanding is opportunity for growth and learning
- Ok to not participate
- Leave space for "weirdness" neurodiversity
- Stimming approved
- Call me by my name

Lessons from the Cup Game Activity:
- Participants reflect on the ice breaker
- Look to young people for solutions
- It's a requirement to meet new people to solve collective problems
- We all took initiative, and there was mutual respect in our initiative

- Allyship–we need to utilize friend's in high places [i.e. the facilitator of the cup game]
- Common ground and common language is important
- Adaptability/flexibility with plans is an asset
- Can't solve the problem alone
- Group thinking is powerful

Building a Restorative Care Practice: What can we use it for? What are necessary ingredients?

- Find out what neighbors need
- Collect contact info in case of emergency
- Safety planning for volatile experiences
- To share Food
- Space to relax that is comfortable, private, familiar, and clean
- Networking and familiarizing
- Ableism—checking it in our self and in the space—how do we hold and confront stigma?
- Skill in holding emotions/co-regulation/self-regulation
- Shared Responsibility

How do we already use Restorative Practice for care?

- Airing grievances
- Solidarity/support [in the work place]
- Sharing food
- Spiritual connection [tarot circle]
- Fellowship
- Trainings
- Networking
- Gathering Info

- Waiting in Public [on Septa, supporting each other during stress]
- Intergenerational connection
- Group therapy/IOP
- Healing circles
- Intimate friendships/kinship
- Recovery circle + food to address political violence [esp. after a protest or action]
- Justice involvement/recovery circles in re-entry/recovery houses
- School mediating fights
- Caregiver/grief support in friend group
- Co-creating community space

Imagined restorative communities:

Participants planned for a restorative community in small groups, and offered their imaginings as a blueprint for future work and next steps. All groups came up with open, accessible third spaces that could be utilized by neighbors in a variety of ways and for a variety of purposes, including to provide safety, to support young people, to share food, and to gather in an emergency.

HOPE Plantation:

- Parks with resources
- Pharmacies with meds
- Place for grief care
- Space to act in madness that is full of compassion
- Arboretum Gardens—refuge full of wildlife, trees, plant, medicine
- Elevators + Escalators, especially for public transit

- Accessible public transit and public spaces, inc ramps, and sidewalks
- Accessible clean water and restrooms
- Libraries
- Somatic bodywork space, sensory deprivation, acupuncture, etc.
- Access to healthy food/including more community gardens growing food

Hirsutim:
- Building culture and expectations
- Healing circles to get away from systems
- Collective Community Garden with labor economy
- Established network to provide resources for elders and single mothers
- Shared safety plan for power grid and energy—storytelling and food during power crisis for whole block to fight isolation
- Appeasing isolation for those with disabilities
- Self-determined youth space with peer connection—autonomy/co-created, older youth lead

OMNI:
- All Ages rec center/community meeting space
- Open 24 hrs, safe place to get resources
- Sports, art, event space, workshops, gated land, tennis courts
- Accessible space wide halls, accessible elevators
- Affordable, accessible

- Community kitchen open late
- Safe for youth, not just centering drinking or spending in order to connect
- Staff is trauma informed

REPRESENT!

Participants of this training represented and shouted out the following organizations:

- Creative Resilient Youth: A youth-led art and mental health advocacy organziation, empowering youth voices + healing via art making + community building, centering BIPOC, LGBTQIA youth interested in learning/discovering more about mental health
- Journey of Hope @ DBHIDS: Journey of Hope offers individuals experiencing prolonged homelessness and behavioral health challenges to embark on a path toward recovery.
- Seed Weed Reap, Aspen Farms Community Garden, and Pearl St. Solidarity Garden: Teaching sustainable agriculture and making herbal medicine accessible to ALL
- Rising Tide Collective @Risingtidephl [IG]: Community of diverse artistic voices sharing resources, audiences + skills
- Morris Home: The only residential recovery program in the country to offer comprehensive services specifically for the transgender community
- People's Environmental Justice Enforcement Agency: Fighting for accountability in environmental justice in Philadelphia
- William Way: Since 1974, William Way has been a resource and hub for the LGBT+ community
- Philly Thrive: Philly Thrive organizes for Environmental Justice!

Offered as a Resource:

- Future Space Philly: Accessible through Philly Suicide Hotline [998]//CIST program is a disability crisis program accessed through crisis line

Suggested learning activities

The following exercise was a part of a workshop entitled Black Muscle Memory: Exploring Black Womxn's Labor (September 2020), developed by the authors for Black Womxn's Time Camp 004, an Afrofuturist workshop series that was a part of an interactive online portal developed and hosted by Black Quantum Futurist Collective during the first year of the COVID-19 pandemic. Black Muscle Memory… challenged participants to engage ancestral memory to access compassion and healing around Black women's labor experiences, especially around care work, domestic work, and organizing in times of civil unrest and racial violence.

Witnessing our bodies' labor stories

Use your labor genogram to find parallels and contrasts between your own bodily experiences in capitalism and their ancestors.

- Take a moment to imagine what labor looked like day to day for any ancestors or family that stick out to you. What images come up for you? Write them below.
- What patterns do you notice about the work and labor patterns that run through your genogram?
- How have you seen those patterns show up for you in your relationship to work today? How do your ancestors live on in your muscle memory?

- How do the effects and spirits of anti-Black capitalism live in you or your family? How have you weaponized capital against other Black people? Or against poor people?

What is My Labor?

- Visualize a near future where daily life has changed because your community has divested from racialized capitalism. Describe your role in this future.

- How does your body feel now that it has been reclaimed from racialized capitalism?

- What are you owed in the present? What is y/our call for reparations and restitution? What can you call for in the present that will lead you to a liberated future?

Surplus persons experience survey: Questions for self and others

The Surplus Persons Experience Survey was first created as part of a multi-media art piece entitled Surplus Persons, done in collaboration with Marcelline Mandeng [audio], Obafemi Matti [visuals], and Cheikh Athj [audio]. This print survey, along with an interactive document of institutionalization was installed for the collaborative art exhibition Time Camp 001 by Black Quantum Futurist Collective at Ice Box Project Space in Philadelphia, PA.

- Have you ever felt expendable? disposable? Unfit for society? Unable to work? Or learn like "normal" people? Have you ever felt left behind? Too sick? Wrong body for forms, wrong body for walking down the street?

- If you have, how do you cope with being a part of the surplus population?

- Do you hide it from coworkers, from partners, from friends? Do you pretend to have resources that you don't have? How often do you do this?

- Do you truly believe you have value in the eyes of your employer? University? High school? therapist's office? Emergency room?

- What makes you feel valuable? If you do not believe you have value, what do you do with that feeling?

- If you are angry, where does it go? If you are envious, where does it go? If you are mournful, where does it go? If you are complacent, where does it go?

- Who do you trust with your feelings of disposability?

- Have you ever given thanks for your invisibility?

- Is there anything to be thankful for in your disposability?

- Do you have a community of disposable or formally disposable people who you can turn to for emotional, political, and economic support?

- Are there times when you feel disposable to your loved ones? Is it because your loved ones struggle with their own disposability? Or because your loved ones have never struggled with disposability?

If you have never felt disposable or been disposed of, what's the closest you have come to expendability?

- Are you friends with any surplus people?

- Do you work with any surplus people?

- Are any of your lovers a part of the surplus population?

- Are you descended from persons who may have been seen as disposable at different points in history?
- Are any of them living?
- Have you spoken to them about their experiences? how does your Family of origin tell your story of familial disposability?
- How often do you push disposable persons from your mind? If they are rarely in your mind, what does it feel like to think of them now?
- Have you ever lived next to a prison? Halfway house? Waste processing plant? Superfund site? Petroleum processing plant? Former lead factory?
- Was it by choice? When you hear of the disposability of others, how do you feel?
  - Are you able to acknowledge how your freedom and/ or wealth is built on the bodies of disposable persons, living and dead?
  - Do you feel an obligation to do so?
  - Do you believe your value is temporary?
- Can you imagine a future where you might be considered disposable? Or a future where currently disposable people are seen as valuable?

Examine your answers for points of intersection and solidarity with others who may encounter overwhelming feelings of helplessness, nihilism, and hopelessness. Examine your answers and experiences for areas of growth, change, and challenge to the status quo that identifies those of us as expendable.

#

The value of local wisdom and history: Discussion questions

In the United States today, scientific and historical facts and information about the lives of marginalized people are put into question, criminalized, and at great risk of erasure, whether from government websites, educational curricula, or in the news media. DSM215 values hyper-local and ancestral wisdom by seeking out and incorporating it from our neighbors and selves into our community practices. We believe by encouraging neighbors to remember and value their community's histories and wisdom, we can find shared truths that reach beyond social media algorithms and elite propaganda and disinformation.

1.   What is your definition of wisdom? How is it different from a winning argument, fact, science, or other concepts of knowledge and knowing.

2.   What sources of wisdom do you value the most? Which sources of wisdom do you struggle to witness or consume?

3.   What histories do you value the most? Which sources of history do you struggle to witness or consume?

4.   What are some examples of local or ancestral wisdom that currently serve you? Describe their impact on you and your practice.

5.   What are some ancestral or familial histories that currently serve you? Describe their impact on you and your practice.

Conclusion

These early years of Deep Space Mind 215's work have been divine and transformative. Time has moved by quickly as we worked to respond organically and directly to our community's needs, leaving little time or space for us to pause, reflect, and document our experiences and the lessons we glean from them. The pursuit of resources to support the work through the non-profit industrial complex added another layer of bureaucracy, urgency, and time scarcity that demands certain results and narratives, without the guarantee of humanization, consistency, or care.

Yet, we, the authors of this book, believe that care workers' experiences addressing global pandemics, complex community issues like homelessness and displacement, and issues of historical trauma are invaluable in the struggle for humanization during Late Capitalism…The pandemic was a clarifying moment for all of the U.S.'s healthcare and social service institutions and systems. Our child welfare, psychiatric, housing, and healthcare infrastructure could not respond to our neighbor's needs the way trusted messengers, mutual aid organizers, and neighborhood sites of care could. Those of us who have lived through these institutions, or with the symptoms, or with disability, were already well versed in this dance of survival and innovation.

This book was not meant to be dogma or a manualized intervention for mental health professionals to roll out at the institutions that employ them. Instead, we trudged through memory, challenge, and experience to model the introspection and intentionality we need in communities across our country.

The antidote to alienation is witnessing real life, felt connection, and regular, life-affirming opportunities to participate in nature and in our own neighborhoods. The antidote to helplessness is community efficacy. It is knowing what neighborhoods deserve and need to thrive. The antidote to disinformation and erasure is intergenerational storytelling and dialogue. The antidote to disillusionment, disbelief, and stagnation is madness, rage, and the pride that comes with accepting the vast neurodiversity within our selves, our ancestry, and our community.

Being tapped into madness is a kind of brilliance that transforms the world; this has always been a collective truth. As we continue to buck against neoliberalism and fascism in the United States, we remain strategic by imagining new ways of being integral parts (individual) of a larger whole (community).

We remember that we're the descendants of Black peoples in the Western hemisphere that have remained in spite of pointed attacks against our personhood, families, and neighborhoods. We remember that we descend from people who have resisted against institutions, against racist laws, and who have lived in spite of grief and death. And that Black madness—the audacity to imagine impossible realities of humanity and joy—is a powerful force worth witnessing and heeding.

We encourage our readers to connect with local wisdom, and with the humanity that comes with accepting madness in ourselves and others. We encourage our readers to persist with those in their communities as we work toward building a new world and to resist the divisions that those in power rely on to continue the eugenicist status quo that continues to threaten our health while new challenges present themselves.

We take heart that offline, in our own backyards, there are neighbors who share the desire to return to each other and to fight for one another's well-being. We believe this power is unstoppable if we are brave enough to seek it out and nurture it.

Notes

1. Igbo landing mass suicide 1803—they chose the sea instead.

2. Guyanese pre-wedding tradition, a large party consisting of the families of the betrothed, complete with food, song, storytelling and jokes about those getting married.

3. Free Application for Federal Student Aid—a heavily flawed bureaucratic process of distributing aid to Americans desiring to attend college, trade school, or any post-secondary training after High School. The FAFSA was revamped under the first Obama administration in an attempt to make the process less burdensome for poor families and more accessible to more Americans.

4. M.O.V.E Bombing at 30: "Barbaric" 1985 Philadelphia Police Attack Killed 11 & Burned a Neighborhood.

5. An upper or ruling class, aristocracy.

6. Tactical Urbanism Movement applies principles of simple, low-cost, and often temporary public space interventions to achieve and accelerate change rather than more expensive long-term equitable interventions. This tactic is commonly used in the process of gentrification.

7. Family Group Conferencing or Family Group Decision making is a form of restorative circle practice adopted by child welfare systems and other family preservation initiatives to support families in collective decision making with their own support system and community, rather than unilateral decisions made by the courts.

8. Area of North Philadelphia comprised of West Oak Lane, Logan, and Fern Rock. Notable sites include Central and Girl's High, the Olney Transportation Center, and Fern Rock Station.

9. *Youth Healers Stand Up!* was a collective of young people with lived experience of homelessness, housing insecurity, and/or systems-involvement who organized for resources and systems-change in the provision of care to homeless youth in Philadelphia. YHSU was active from [date to date] and had a hand.

Bibliography

Brown, N., Jenks, A., Nelson, K., and Tilghman, L. (2020). *Teaching COVID-19: An Anthropology Syllabus Project*. Teaching and Learning Anthropology. Available at: https://docs.google.com/document/u/0/d/1-IRVbz1nsBQJHcaCVh8QLRBiwj3cFT_bXSwm TNs_Hf0/mobilebasic

Bruce, L. J. (2021). *How to Go Mad without Losing Your Mind: Madness and Black Radical Creativity*. Duke University Press.

Cutlass Mashramani, R. (2016). A Young Thug Confronts His Own Future. In *Style of Attack Report*. Metropolarity. Available at: https://metropolarity.net/2015/08/a-young-thug-confronts-his-own-future/

Cutlass, R. M. (2017). *Surplus Person Questions for Persons at Risk* [Print Publication, Installation]. Black Quantum Futurist Collective Time Camp 001. Available at: https://www.blackwomentempo ral.net/surpluspersons

Daniels, B. (2023). *Journal of a Black Queer Nurse*. Common Notions.

Deep Space Mind 215. (2024.). *Deep Space Mind 215 Website*. DSM214. Available at: www.deepspacemind215.com

Disempower, Disarm, Disband. (2024). *A World without Police*. Available at: http://aworldwithoutpolice.org/

Division of Clinical Psychology. (2018). *Power Threat Meaning— Full Version* (p. bpsrep.2018.inf299b). British Psychological Society. Available at: https://doi.org/10.53841/bpsrep.2018.inf299b

Dixon, E., and Piepzna-Samarasinha, L. L. (2020). *Beyond Survival: Strategies and Stories from the Transformative Justice Movement*. AK Press.

Dukmasova, M. (2016). Abolish the Police? Organizers Say It's Less Crazy Than It Sounds. *The Chicago Reader*. Available at: https://chicagoreader.com/news-politics/abolish-the-police-organizers-say-its-less-crazy-than-it-sound

Evains, T. S. (2022, May 2). *Alondra Park, El Camino College Replaced a Planned Luxury Black Neighborhood Called "Gordon Manor."* Available at: https://www.dailybreeze.com/2022/05/02/alondra-park-el-camino-college-replaced-a-planned-luxury-black-neighborhood-called-gordon-manor/

Faroul, R. (2021). Philadelphia Renters Report: COVID-19's Impact on Race and Housing Security Across Philadelphia. *Community Legal Services*. Available at: https://clsphila.org/wp-content/uploads/2021/02/20210222-Philadelphia-Renters-Report.pdf

Fattah, Q. M. F. (Ed.). (2024). *Umoja Magazine*. House of Umoja Magazine. https://www.houseofumoja.net/umojamagazine.html

Fontaine, F. G. (1861). American Abolition 1787 to 1861. *Library of Congress*. Available at: https://drive.google.com/file/d/1-4aVnRafj12yu--YeDstJgto2EnXBLZF/view?usp=sharing

Freire, P. (2017). *Pedagogy of the Oppressed*. Penguin Classics.

Fullilove, M. T. (2016). *Root Shock: How Tearing Up City Neighborhoods Hurts America, and What We Can Do about It*. Fullilove, M. T. Available at: https://doi.org/10.2307/j.ctt21pxmmc

Given, M. (2021, July 21). *Two Organizations Collaborate for an Important Conversation through Art*. Available at: https://metrophiladelphia.com/two-organizations-collaborate-for-an-important-conversation-through-art/

Hazzard, K. (2022). *American Sirens*. Hatchett Books.

Hersey, T. (2022). *Rest Is Resistance: A Manifesto*. Little Brown Spark.

Hill-Jarrett, T. G. (2023). The Black Radical Imagination: A Space of Hope and Possible Futures. *Frontiers in Neurology*, 14, 1241922. Available at: https://doi.org/10.3389/fneur.2023.1241922

Ilunga, M., and Ilunga, K. (2020). *Canned Responses for Black People*. Hastag Protect Your Energy. Available at: https://hashtagprotec tyourenergy.weebly.com

Jacobs, J. (2016). The city lament genre in the ancient Near East. *The fall of cities in the Mediterranean (commemoration in literature, folk-song, and liturgy)*, 13–32.

Jones, K., and Okun, T. (2001). *White Supremacy Culture* [Workshop]. Available at: https://www.cwsworkshop.org/PARC_site_B/dr-cult ure.html

Jovenes Inc. (2023). Los Padrinos, Jovenes Website. *Jovenes Website*. Available at: https://jovenesinc.org/newsite/los-padrinos/

Lipsky, L. v, and Burk, C. (2009). *Trauma Stewardship: An Everyday Guide to Caring for Self while Caring for Others*. Berrett-Koehler Publisher, Inc.

McCartney, R., and Belknap, T. (2017). *Distance=/=Time: An Immersive Multimedia Exhibition Investigating Relationships of Science and Self*. Icebox Project Space.

Mitani, H., Kondo, N., and Tabuchi, T. (2024). Promotive and Protective Effects of Community-Related Positive Childhood Experiences on Adult Health Outcomes in the Context of Adverse Childhood Experiences: A Nationwide Cross-Sectional Survey in Japan. BMJ Open.

Nopper, T. K. (2021). *Anti-Asian Violence and Black-Asian Solidarity Today* [Lecture]. Asian American Writers' Workshop, Online. Available at: https://youtu.be/MGpo9419ViE

Ortiz, L., and Jani, J. (2010). Critical Race Theory: A Transformational Model for Teaching Diversity. *Journal of Social Work Education*, 46(2), pp. 175–193. Available at: https://doi.org/10.5175/ JSWE.2010.200900070

Page, C., and Woodland, E. (2023). *Healing Justice Lineages: Dreaming at the Crossroads of Liberation, Collective Care, and Safety*. North Atlantic Books.

Philips, R. (2020). *Community Futurisms: Space Time Collapse: Vol. II.* House of Future Sciences Books.

Philips, R. (2022). Colonized Time, Racial Time, and the Legal Time of Progress. *Poverty Race and Research Action Council*, 31(1).

Philips, R. (2025). *Dismantling the Master's Clock: On Race, Space, and Time.* AK Press.

Philly Folklore Project (Director). (Filmed 1991. Digital Upload 2015). *Blanche Epps In the Garden of Gethsemane* [Archival Interview. Film.]. Available at: https://youtu.be/QegjoDMk ShQ?si=dkqFOQF1f3ojOmlJ

Pickens, A. T. (2019). *Black Madness: Mad Blackness.* Duke University Press.

Piepzna-Samarasinha, L. L. (2022). *The Future Is Disabled: Prophecies, Love Notes, Mourning Songs.* Arsenal Pulp Press.

Pirtle Laster, W. N. (2020). Racial Capitalism: A Fundamental Cause of Novel Coronavirus. *Health, Education and Behavior*, 1(5), pp. 1–5.

Pulido, L. (2016). Flint, Environmental Racism, and Racial Capitalism. *Capitalism Nature Socialism*, 27(3), pp. 1–16. Available at: https://doi.org/10.1080/10455752.2016.1213013

Rauch, T. (2021). *Roots before Branches.* Available at: https://yout ube.com/watch?v=EEUFb338hHg

Shange, Ntozake. (1997). *For Colored Girls Who Have Considered Suicide, When the Rainbow Is enuf. Scribner, 1997.* Scribner.

Stanford, R. (2022). Intergenerational Partnerships Can Curb Youth Violence. *The Appeal.* Available at: https://theappeal.org/intergenerational-partnerships-can-curb-gun-violence/

West Philly Local. (2012, December 24). *Fire Destroy's Elena's Soul.* Available at: https://www.westphillylocal.com/2012/12/24/fire-destroys-elenas-sou

WHYY. (n.d.). *Bhutan's Happiness Measurement Model* [Broadcast]. Available at: https://whyy.org/episodes/beyond-measure

Wilderson, F. B. (2020). *Afropessimism* (First edition). Liveright Publishing Corporation.

Zimbardo, P., Sword, R., and Sword, R. (2012). *Time Cure: Overcoming PTSD with the New Psychology of Time Perspective Therapy*. Jossey-Bass Books.

Further reading

Rashni's recommendations

Philips, R. (2020). *Community Futurisms: Space-time Collapse II*. House of Future Sciences Books.

Piepzna-Samarasinha, L. L. (2022). *The Future Is Disabled: Prophecies, Love Notes, Mourning Songs*. Arsenal Pulp Press.

Cutlass, R. (2016). "A Young Thug Confronts His Own Future."

Philips, R. (2025). *Dismantling the Master's Clock: On Race, Space, and Time*. AK Press.

Philips, R. (2022). *Colonized Time, Racial Time, and the Legal Time of Progress*. Poverty Race and Research Action Council.

Cutlass, R. (2017). Surplus persons, digital installation with Marcelline Mandeng, Femi Matti and Cheikh Ath, Time Camp 001 with Black Quantum Futurism, Oct 2017. Available at: www.blackwomentemporal.net/surpluspersons.

Dixon, E., and Piepzna-Samarasinha, L. L. (2020). *Beyond Survival: Strategies and Stories from the Transformative Justice Movement*. AK Press.

Lipsky, L. v, and Burk, C. (2009). *Trauma Stewardship: An Everyday Guide to Caring for Self While Caring for Others*. Berrett-Koehler Publisher, Inc.

#

Mel's further reading recommendations

Bambara, T. C. (2017). *Conversations with Toni Cade Bambara*. Literary Conversations.

Freire, P. (2017). *Pedagogy of the Oppressed*. Penguin Classics.

O'Brien, M. E., & Abdelhadi, E. (2022). An oral history of the New York Commune: 2052-2072.

Wilderson, F. B. (2020). *Afropessimism* (First edition). Liveright Publishing Corporation.

About the authors

Mel Bunni Brown

I spent my formative years in the Bay Area, shoreside is where I learned to tell stories, saw my first black widow in her web at the foot of an eucalyptus tree. Learning the importance of Black resistance and collective struggle. I spent summers sleeping underneath redwoods. Even in my deep affections for the west coast, I'd consider the midwesterner city of Saint Louis as where I grew up. Watching the rise and fall of the mississippi river, learning about grief, the sweetness of peach custard ice cream from Iggy's Ice Cream shop, and digging up clay banks of the meramec river.

Philadelphia accepted my call for adventure, taught me how to organize with youth, gave me battle scars, showed me that I was enough. It is an honor to hold Philly's history of long forgotten times, learning how to pack light, being nomadic, and flexible. I've collected memories of the long lines at Fred's water ice, finding shade underneath the Belmont plateau tree while dirt bikes circle the fields, taking my kids to cooled off in the devil's pool of the Wissahickon, remembering the sadness and ash that christmas eve air carried the day Elena's Soul on 49th & Baltimore burned down. Philadelphia is my home, which beckoned me, to it— through the words of the poets, song writers, and those stricken with madness.

Rashni Stanford

I have been in Philadelphia now for 20 years. This has been the most stable home I have ever had, something the younger versions of me still struggle to digest and understand. I came here at 17 years old, unaccompanied and unsupported. I became estranged from my family of origin for over a decade while I continued the task of growing up under the auspices of this city. I have been hospitalized three times here, parented and mentored so many children and young people. I've partied here, watched lovers come and go from this place.

The ways Philadelphia has adopted me have shown themselves not only in the acceptance and care I have received from neighbors and co-patients in institutions during my lowest points but also in the ways my ideas have been able to grow under collective nurturance and encouragement. The city and its people have always been clear with me about its boundaries, limits, and its interests and joys. I realize so many transplants have not had the divine privilege of this intimate love, and I cherish every child's birthday cake, baby shower meatball shared with me, and every crab broken in solidarity on the stoop.

I thank every coworker or neighbor who showed themselves as loving guides and elders for me as I showed my ass as a young person, who gathered me with care and clarity, and built trust in me with their honesty and directness.

I remember at 20 years old, finally getting hired as a domestic violence hotline worker, and attending my first staff meeting with five new coworkers, all of whom were over the age of 45. One of them cocked her eyebrow at me and crossed her arms, "What makes you think you can do this work?" Our white supervisor bristled with embarrassment and anxiety, while I relished the authenticity.

"Well Miss, I'm not gonna waste time trying to convince you, but I promise to show you the kind of worker I am." And I did.

I have immense gratitude for all the Philadelphians who met me in that authenticity in all capacities I have inhabited as community practitioner. To my roommates in psychiatric institutions, and the staff who managed me at my most dissociated and rageful. To the renters who participated in the focus groups for the Philadelphia Renters Report research project during the onset of the COVID-19 pandemic, and their searing honesty and support for one another during those Zoom sessions (Faroul, 2021; Philips, 2022). To the youth that built *Youth Healers Stand Up!*[9] with me, and all of the youth-led policies and norms they fought relentlessly for, despite their own housing and wellness challenges. To all the neighbors, hummingbirds, and groundhogs who visited Pentridge Children's Garden this summer, and their willingness to embrace possibility and change as a collective. To all the nerds, punks, spiritual leaders, writers, and artists who have created alongside me and have come to form my family in Afrofuturist practice—to Metropolarity, Black Quantum Futurist Collective, and Community Futures Lab. To the Lenape people, and their ancestors throughout Lenapehoking whose ancestral practices and blessings have made a way for me as a thrown-away teen in North Jersey, and a whole adult down here in the Delaware Valley.

Thank you for raising me, and keeping me. And I hope these words do justice to the power we all share as we inhabit this land together.

\#

Index

www.ingramcontent.com/pod-product-compliance
Lightning Source LLC
Chambersburg PA
CBHW070346270326
41926CB00017B/4010